Reviews

"Transformation Road" takes the reader on the long and often tragic journey of Sean Anderson's battle with food and morbid obesity spanning just about his entire life. His experience with declaring war with himself graphically depicts the tortured soul of most of us who face an addictive and pathological relationship with food. Having won many a battle but inevitably losing his war, Sean offers us some insight as to who the real enemy has been.

To be sure, compulsive eating, binge eating, and the many "flavors" of related forms of food addiction and eating disorders [e.g. bulimia, anorexia] do not all lend themselves to a "one size fits all" solution. However, there does seem to be a common thread among those, like Sean, who find their way to recovery- namely rigorous self-honesty, an open mind, and, as Sean would remind us, an "iron-clad" willingness to change.

"Transformation Road" takes the reader away from the typical weight loss fixes and asks the reader to consider the nature of emotional eating and the "symptom" of obesity. The author reveals his "moment of clarity" and the resultant decision to declare a truce with his war with food. What follows is Sean's recipe for food addiction recovery. Although incorporating some suggestions that run contrary to some recovered food addicts, Sean's experiences are worth learning about and considering.

As someone who has worked with patients suffering with all forms of eating disorders for more than three decades, I think Sean's book is a must read for anyone touched by the effects of food addiction and obesity. More important than his weight loss is his ability to testify to the basic tenets of recovery from any addiction- namely honesty, open mindedness, and willingness. In some recovery circles this is known by an acronym H.O.W.

Marty Lerner, PhD.
CEO, Milestones In Recovery
Eating Disorders Program

"Don't think of this as a weight loss book. This book is for anyone who has ever battled themselves, in other words, it's for all of us. I believe we are all born broken and the only thing separating us is the individual routes we take away from, or toward wholeness. Sean's journey is laid out for you here with all of it's twists, turns, false starts, dead ends, and breakthroughs. Although the paths you and I travel may be different, I am certain that you, like me, will recognize many of the stops and ultimately gain insight into yourself through Sean's journey. I enthusiastically recommend this book, not for Sean's miraculous outer changes, but for his ability to take you on the inside, where real transformation must always happen."

Dave May
"Mayday In The Morning"-KLOR

"Sean Anderson provides a strong dose of hope in recounting his captivating journey to self-acceptance and health. His road to transformation was not easy, but few things in life are that are worth it. Sean reminds us that your biggest bully is often yourself and that you can change your "mix tape in your head" by becoming your own "captain." This book demonstrates that the only thing that can make us feel good about ourselves is to realize our own self-worth, and to finally love ourselves. I constantly see patients struggling to make the mental shift required to commit to change and make good choices for their health. Whether you are struggling with weight loss, addiction, and self-acceptance or whether you are just looking to be inspired to finally commit to change and making good choices – this is the book for you."

Dr. Amy Cox
The Ranch Chiropractic Wellness Center

"Reading Sean's story has given me a window on the day-to-day realities of a life ruled by food. I admire the courage he shows by revealing intimate details of his life, not sparing himself, not blaming others, and respecting the dignity of others. With the creation of his simple yet profound "Calorie Bank and Trust" concept, Sean provided himself a means to accomplish genuine, sustainable weight loss when all his previous attempts had failed. I am eager to introduce my customers to the inspiring story of this man of extraordinary insight, determination, and compassion."

Jean Brace
Brace Books & More

"Sean's book is so good that I pretty much read it in two sittings. If I had the time, I would have read the entire thing in one sitting. I related to his story on so many levels, and I believe any morbidly obese person will. I really, really want to share so much from the book, but I want you to buy the book. I know I will when it comes out. I'm actually going to buy a few copies, and when I see someone struggling with weight loss, I'm going to give them a copy because someone (Sean) has finally put into words the secret of weight loss. First off, there is no secret. We all know that. Second, Sean really dives into the mental aspects of weight loss and the journey. We all know about watching calorie levels and exercising.... but he gets into the mental aspect of weight loss, which is critical to success...His book is the best weight loss book that I've ever read. No other book goes into the mental aspect of weight loss quite like his book does."

Stephen Vinson
whoatemyblog.com

"With Transformation Road, Sean Anderson delivers a riveting story of a man who faced death and won. Amazingly, this isn't your typical murder mystery- it's Sean's true battle against a lethal killer - morbid obesity. For the millions who have lost faith in ever beating their own war with food, Transformation Road offers hope and inspiration."

Gerri Helms, MCC, CSC
Author, "Trust God and Buy Broccoli, a Spiritual Approach to Weight Loss"
www.lifecoachgerri.com

"He lost the weight and salvaged his future, doing it without pills, without a big-name program and without salads. He looked into the abyss of his own terrifying food addiction and he slowly backed away, blogging every step of the way. I've spent much of my life morbidly obese, and though I never tipped the scales near Sean's heaviest, I can relate to the feeling of hopelessness and helplessness that comes across here. I think anyone who's ever stared intently at the bathroom mirror on a Monday morning and proclaimed "This is it!" will as well. "Transformation Road" is the story of redemption, reclamation, and salvation. Weight loss is the ultimate 'do-it-yourself project', and Sean Anderson shares the blueprints and tools you need to build a happier, healthier future."

Jack Sh*t
Healthy Living Blogger

"When I started to read "Transformation Road" I could not stop. I finished it in a couple of days. All thirty plus chapters of it. There were so many times I laughed....and a couple of times I cried. This book is amazing. It could possibly be one of the most helpful books for weight loss. It does not say you have to lose weight like this or give you a detailed explanation of how he did it. It gives you the "Whys" of Sean's life. It is amazing that Sean is a success story for weight loss when years before, he wanted to be a success story for other things. I have been overweight for most of my life and I have read hundreds of weight loss and inspirational books. Sean's book is the only book I have read that showed me the selfishness I have had with food, and the true importance of losing weight. No fad diet, just a story to tell."

Tony Posnanski --221 pound loser.

Transformation Road

My Trip to Over 500 Pounds and Back

Sean A. Anderson

www.TotalPublishingAndMedia.com

Cover Photo: Reflections By Brittany Combs and Katrina Cope
Back Cover Author's Photo: Darryl Cox
Various photo credits within: Kelli Anderson
Cover design: Christina Rich-Splawn
580-716-5446
x-tina@grafxtina.com

ISBN: 978-1-937829-12-4

Dedicated to the loving memory of my little brother, David Shane Anderson.

You're always with me.

Acknowledgments

I t all started with simply sharing my thoughts, fears, desires, experiences, and absolute determination to succeed at losing weight every day on my weight loss blog. The commitment required an investment of time and emotional energy. As I began to unravel my history of food addiction and compulsive or emotional eating, I started to get down to my very core, where suddenly, I could clearly see exactly how I was keeping myself imprisoned. Then, like I was given the key to my own cell, I was able to clearly see the way out, for me. And it has been a glorious liberation.

I believe it was Irene, my wife of twenty-one years, who first suggested I would eventually write a book. And then several like suggestions would follow, occasionally showing up in the comments left on my blog, by those who were also discovering the power they had to set themselves free. Each suggestion would give me confidence, until eventually it was decided. I would write this book. But not *this* book. No, I had something very different in mind, something much easier. The idea, suggested by some loyal readers of my blog, was to simply turn my blog into some kind of daily inspirational. And it could still happen. Maybe the book could be the first three hundred sixty-five days, heavily edited down, and I could provide present-day commentary with hindsight over each entry. But no, that is not *this book.*

What you're now holding in your hand is something very different from the pages of The Daily Diary of a Winning Loser. This is my life story. Perhaps it seems a little premature to write such a memoir at thirty-nine years old. But it makes perfect sense. It does, because my life will forever be divided into several sections, with two very different versions of me. If I ever write another, perhaps it will cover age forty, onward. I must live it first. And that's exactly what I've done in these pages. Lived it and learned from it, and taken a bunch of family and friends along for the ride.

The incredible support I've been given from my family and friends is simply an amazing blessing. The sacrifices along this road have been many and certainly not just endured by me, but by everyone around me, who despite it all, loves me regardless of anything and everything. I've been given a gift of love from so many, who gave it long before I ever started transforming. And it's that love, regardless of my size and appearance or the crazy twist and turns I created along the way, that has never been jeopardized, because it's unconditional, based on love in its purest, most perfect form.

Irene, along with our daughters Amber and Courtney, experienced much of this story first hand, as did my mom, who obviously has been along from day one. Their support, along with loving support from my dear grandma, Aunt Kelli, Uncle Keith, my late grandpa, and little brother Shane, combined to make my foundation exactly what it became. A tight-knit family unit, where different struggles may have always played a role, but never changed the love we had for one another.

Many people came together to help make this project come to life. My cousin Sherri Finch really stepped in at a perfect time, counseling me and challenging me to look at my opportunities from a different perspective. Her business and entrepreneurial sense is sharply tuned and level. Her business prowess has helped build her company, Finch Insurance Services, into a solid and successful company, and now, she lends her support and talents to seeing this project blossom into reality.

When I eventually realized what a major undertaking a book like this could become, I must admit, I was a little unsure of myself. Gerri Helms, a published author herself, and a certified master life coach, signed on to be my life coach at exactly the perfect time. Her insight into the dynamics involved along the way and her always positive encouragement, combined with constructive challenges, taught me a great deal. Not just about writing a book, but about being accountable to oneself, and moving forward, one step at a time, slowly but surely. Her personal triumph over her own food addiction and obesity, with nearly twenty years of maintenance behind her, gave me a tremendous bonus. I learned a powerful lesson in the differences that make each of our journeys unique. At the end of the day, the fundamental dynamics of addiction may be the same, but how we overcome can vary slightly from person to person. The results and joy that engulf our lives are relative to our experiences, expectations, individual taste, and desires. And we overcome and accomplish beautifully in our own unique and glorious way.

Peter Biadasz of Total Publishing and Media has authored over sixteen books and been credited with helping many more first-time authors through the publishing process. His gift of sitting me down and giving me a crash course of what a new author can expect in the publishing world was full of hard truths, straightforward advice, and positive encouragement. Some of the things he told me were disappointing, because I was ready to become a full-time writer *from page one.* But his honest portrayal of what it meant and required was sobering, yet invaluable to understand and process. And when the literary critique of my work included things I didn't want to read or accept, he patiently understood my response and countered with solid advice and reasoning.

The discipline required to finally finish this book was encouraged through many long months by several people, namely Karen Burghardt. I swear, she must have thought I would never really be done. I would often spend hours staring blankly at the screen, analyzing every little detail, rereading over and over, and revising. Karen was always understanding and ready to offer her ear and opinion. It was like having an editor standing by, ready to process chapter by chapter, paragraph by paragraph, and sometimes word by word. I can be extremely critical of myself and message, not too much on content, but how it's communicated. So yes, sometimes, word by word. Her often times instant feedback was always helpful.

When I finally finished the manuscript, I consulted a colleague about some of the chapter and section titles. What happened from there, wasn't what I thought I wanted, but ended up being an incredible enhancement to this work. I was finished and happy to be finished. But Dave May challenged me to go a little further, dig a little deeper, and really give a more complete understanding of the overall message within these pages. I resisted at first, but as I read my words to Dave, he clearly was identifying with the road I had traveled through the clutches of addiction. His insight and offerings were golden and on point with every suggestion. His wisdom enhanced my own understanding and played a wonderful role in helping me convey the messages and emotions I was determined to share. Every manuscript needs a rewrite and the extra time and care taken to accomplish this phase, I believe, was a tremendous gift to me.

The patience extended me from numerous others, throughout the writing of this book, including my boss at Team Radio, Bill Coleman, and co-worker Gayle Williams, was at times, exhausting—I'm sure. I was given an amazing amount of understanding, encouragement, and time, to get this book finished. The good-natured humor revolving around the expected completion dates along the way, never became stale. They knew it would eventually get done, when at times, it seemed to never end. Kind of like this list of acknowledgments.

Thank you to all I've mentioned here, and to you, for reading what I hope you'll find to be well worth your investment. I also owe a huge debt of gratitude to the wonderful readers of my weight loss blog. Your support, understanding, advice, and encouragement from day one, along with the critical element of accountability you provided, have given me the strength to accomplish what I once thought impossible.

I was surely going to die young, a victim of morbid obesity, because I felt powerless to my addiction. But I now know, real change is possible—even for someone as lost as I once was. I'm found and wonderfully alive. And I give thanks to God for every personal epiphany and revelation discovered along the way. My hope is, I've conveyed my message, communicated in a way that will make an impact for anyone who desires positive change.

I'm honored to have one of my writing heroes, Ralph Marston JR., contribute the foreword to this book. Mr. Marston writes with a clarity so real and truthful, you would have a hard time finding anyone to disagree with his motivating messages. His writing has been and continues to be a major blessing to me and so many others around the World. I'm so thankful to my dear cousin Debbie Hadley for introducing me to his work, early in my transformation.

Thank you again for your wonderful support. My best to you always.

Good Choices,
Sean A. Anderson

Contents

Foreword

L ife is all about choices. Often, it doesn't seem that way, though. We regularly fool ourselves into thinking that the life we experience is imposed on us from the outside, and is the result of factors beyond our control. It's easy and even comforting to think of ourselves as victims, because that relieves us of the burden of responsibility.

The problem is, such thinking is a tragic deception. For decades, Sean Anderson lied to himself in this manner. He told himself that food was the enemy. It seemed a perfectly reasonable thing to assume, because he was eating so much food he became morbidly obese. But the food was never the problem. The problem lay entirely in Sean's choices.

Life is all about choices, and the bad news is that we cannot ever successfully escape from that responsibility. But there's good news, too, and it is much more powerful and potent than the bad news. The good news is that our choices give us control over our lives. When we choose to exercise that control, anything is possible.

This book is a true story about two people. They both have the same name, the same personality, the same likes and dislikes, the same life dreams, skills and passions. In fact, they both occupy the same identity. These two people are separated only by time, and most importantly, by choices. The first person is Sean, before he makes the decision to take responsibility for his choices. He is masterful at coping with his obesity and other challenges, and yet is even more skilled at ignoring the fundamental cause of his problems and at excusing his own poor choices. Many of those excuses you'll find to be very familiar. I know I did.

The other main character in this story is also Sean, after he makes the commitment to take positive control of his life and his health. This is the truly inspiring person, who fully embraces his responsibility. He finds great joy and fulfillment in the positive choices he makes, and eagerly shares his story of transformation with others.

When someone sheds more than fifty percent of his body weight, that is quite a transformation. Yet the real transformation here has nothing to do with pounds lost or waistline measurements or calories consumed. The real substance of Sean Anderson's transformation came in an instant, when he made the authentic and non-negotiable commitment to take complete responsibility for his own life. Once that happened, his weight loss and all the other good things associated with it could not help but occur. The inner transformation happened immediately. The outward manifestation of that transformation began to follow just as surely as day follows night, and will continue indefinitely. That's not to say that it was easy for Sean to lose so much weight, or that it will ever be easy to keep it off. It takes an impressive level of discipline to achieve what he has achieved. It is that inner commitment, that inner transformation, from which the discipline surely and steadily flows.

Sean's life up to this point has been an amazing journey, and he has now created an even brighter future for himself by virtue of the choices he has made. In recounting this story, he very generously and openly acknowledges a long list of shortcomings and insecurities, some of them quite intimate. That makes it all the more powerful and inspiring. After all, we each have worries, doubts and vulnerabilities that we often try to hide even from ourselves. And just as with most political scandals, the cover-up does more damage than the underlying issue. It's wonderfully refreshing and inspiring to see what can happen when someone steps away from the excuses, lets go of the rationalizations, stops choosing to be a victim, and makes the commitment to make a positive difference.

Truth is powerful. The more you seek to hide from it, the more forcefully it asserts itself, until you eventually cannot deny it. The moment you put truth on your side, all sorts of positive possibilities open up to you. That's what Sean Anderson chose to do, and it's a choice that has turned his life around in a dramatic and inspiring way. It's a choice available to anyone, from any background, in any situation, no matter what has or has not happened before. No special skill or complicated training is needed to put your life on the side of truth. All it takes is the desire to live an authentic life of meaning and fulfillment. This story is a compelling and unforgettable reminder that the best choice is always yours to make, no matter what.

Ralph Marston
The Daily Motivator
www.GreatDay.com

.

Chapter 505

Prelude with the Author

If you've read from page one, then you've covered the reviews (I'm very thankful for these wonderful words!), acknowledgments (I hope I didn't leave anyone out), and an amazing foreword by Ralph Marston. *Ralph Marston, The Daily Motivator, in my book, can you believe that?*

But before you go any further, I just wanted to say something. Let's pretend the two of us have run into one another and you've informed me you're getting ready to read my book. If we spent a few minutes discussing what you're about to read, here's what I would say:

This isn't a typical how-to type of weight loss book. I spent my childhood growing into the habits and behaviors contributing to my morbid obesity, and then I spent nearly twenty years of adulthood—near, at, or above 500 pounds. To better understand the dynamics involved, it was necessary to start at the beginning. This analytical exploration has been a critical element in embracing my personal truth and was what I needed to do in order to really break free. Again, this isn't a typical weight loss book.

If you want, you could skip to the last part of the book and experience more of a how-to type of explanation. But something important to remember is this: To fully understand the philosophies and approach that worked for me, the entire story is relevant. It is my story, my methods, my way. And you may or may not relate to or find my approach to be doable for you, and that's fine. We're all different, yet the same in many ways. One thing is certain, there are many successful paths to freedom. In this book, you just might find some similarities between us. And in those similarities, you could possibly gain clarity toward your own road out of whatever is holding you back from what you truly desire.

You may have found this book listed under "weight loss," or "self-help," or "health," because it's about me and my experiences. But it's not only about weight loss. The recipe for freedom from my food addiction and compulsive or emotional eating, and the resulting obesity, is a recipe that can be adapted to fit you and your situation. When I speak or write about *"choosing change before change chooses you,"* it's certainly not exclusively about weight loss. It's about living the life you passionately desire and making the choices that put you in the best position to achieve those dreams.

I've always been a dreamer and I've always been fascinated by irony. In my wildest dreams, I never once imagined my morbidly obese life could be turned inside out, and now, the very thing determined to kill me, has transformed into a passionate desire to spend the rest of my life shining a light on a road many of us travel.

Thank you for taking the time to read the next thirty-six chapters. I hope you'll share your thoughts with me afterward when we run into one another again. Or just send me an email to sean@transformationroad.com

Are you ready? The next exit is chapter one. Happy travels. . .

Sean A. Anderson

Section One

Building the Cell

"How I became a food addict, one choice at a time."

Chapter One

Born Hungry

From all accounts, it was a difficult delivery for this young lady of twenty-six. A small framed woman, four foot eleven, and in labor for the first time. She was scared and alone. This wasn't how it was supposed to happen. The hopes and dreams for this new chapter were very different not long before this day. Fragments of a broken relationship preceded what was sure to be one of the most physically painful experiences of Beverly Anderson's life. The circumstances weren't perfect, but life wasn't waiting for perfect. It was quickly moving forward and Beverly was tightly holding on.

With a firm grip of a family member's hand, this young woman lovingly accepted the pain that would deliver her son into the world. The doctor had reason to be concerned because this wasn't a routine delivery. The baby was a little larger than average and this young woman was a little smaller than most. At 10:06 PM on October 23rd, 1971, this big baby boy, after a difficult birth, laid in his momma's arms with his little right arm, motionless, perhaps somehow damaged in the process, but otherwise the picture of health at nine pounds five ounces. Meet Sean Allen Anderson, that's me, I'm that big bundle of joy. But I don't really remember much until a little while later. And then, *oh man,* I remember all kinds of things, like my first vivid memory of food.

I like it thin and crispy, easy on the sauce, with extra cheese. The aroma in the parking lot of Ken's Pizza Parlor increased the excited anticipation of the feast to come. Walking inside and absorbing the smells and atmosphere of this place was something I had been buzzing about for awhile. Watching the perfect circles of heaven as they made their way out of the oven via the conveyor rack was fascinating too. Everyone was smiling at me, everyone came bearing gifts, and everyone came hungry. The cake was, well, honestly—I don't remember much about the cake. I'm sure it was a custom-baked creation from the IGA grocery store bakery. No, I was focused on getting my fill of pizza and soda pop. There was nothing abnormal about the scene, not in the least. It was a celebration, a perfect one if you ask me, full of happy people—family, friends, gifts, party hats, and plenty of food, *glorious food.* And a drum set, a brand new drum set—I almost forgot. My attention was pulled in a tug of war between the gifts and the food, *but mostly the food.* It was a perfect recipe for comfort and happiness, and it wouldn't have been the same without all of the fantastic elements that made my fourth birthday party so memorable.

I started finding comfort in food at four years old. I wouldn't fully realize it until over thirty years later, but even as a young child, that emotional dependency was there. I was always bigger than the other kids, I wasn't necessarily obese. No, we had friendlier words, like "husky." So, I was a *husky* child, not grotesquely obese yet—just big enough to be different. Big enough for Mark Peterson to know, that if he wanted to secure his reputation as someone you didn't pick on, he needed to make a statement on my first day of kindergarten at Pleasant View Elementary. Lunchtime couldn't come fast enough. I needed some peanut butter and jelly comfort, and an extra helping, *please.*

I started kindergarten at Westwood Elementary two months prior to my first day at Pleasant View. The first day at Westwood wasn't bad at all, I mean, it was everyone's first day—nobody was bold enough to make any kind of statement. We were all just trying hard not to pee ourselves. My *second* first day of kindergarten was brought about by a careless smoker next door from us in our little one-bedroom duplex. It was just Mom and me living in this small place, or "cozy" place, as Mom liked to say, when one night the smoker next door decided it was a great idea to smoke in bed.

The fire raged through our little home, but we didn't wake, no— we were fast asleep when it all came burning down. For some strange reason, even Mom can't really say why, on the night of the fire, we decided to stay at grandma and grandpa's house, a mere mile or so from our cozy little fire-gutted duplex.

We needed a place to live, and Southern Heights, the government-subsidized apartments on the Southern edge of Stillwater, had an immediate opening. Southern Heights was conveniently located directly across the street from a little independent school known as Pleasant View—the place where my early childhood behaviors would develop and where my defining experiences would happen. It was a place that despite the name, really didn't have a pleasant view of anything. At least, not from the perspective of a five-year-old Sean Anderson.

With Mom I felt safe, I was protected by this strong single parent, who, if she was scared, never showed it to me. When she walked me into Mrs. Hesser's kindergarten class on that cool October morning, I didn't want her to leave, *ever*. I reluctantly shuffled into the room and looked at my new classmates with a timid-fearful expression. Mom knew I was nervous, and did her best to comfort me with her soothing voice, but she could have talked all day. The only thing that would have worked was if they enrolled her too. I hadn't been assigned a seat, so I was instructed to sit in a chair alongside the teacher's desk, facing the class, and facing my mom, who by now, realized that I was frightened. She looked at me with calm, reassuring me that everything was going to be fine, and she would pick me up at noon. Mom turned to leave the class and at the same time, so did Mrs. Hesser.

I was sitting all alone in a class full of five-year-olds. The look of fear coming from me, a husky little boy, must have sent some kind of signal to Mark Peterson, who was rather small for his age. In fact, he was the smallest kid in the class. Mark decided, as soon as the coast was clear with the adults out of the room, that he was going to send a message to every impressionable *kindergärtner* in attendance. Mark got up out of his little chair and walked up to me like he was doing his

5

best impression of Clint Eastwood. Not a word was said, just a look. He sized me up within seconds and realized that I was scared to death, and that's when he unleashed an unprovoked and surprisingly powerful kick to my shin. Mark Peterson wasn't going to be picked on because he was small, and now, everyone knew it . . . but as I crumbled to the floor in frightened tears, they also knew, that despite my larger size, I would never fight back. They knew I was a soft-hearted peace lover. They knew I was a big, *easy target.*

For the next several weeks, every time Mrs. Hesser would leave the room, I would cry, and Tina King would comfort me. *"It'll be alright, Sean, you're going to be alright,"* she would say, and I believed her. It was the beginning of what I later realized was my "internal hope mechanism." We later exchanged phone numbers and became a first-grade couple. It was cute. She would call me and I would call her. I wish I could remember what we, as two first graders, actually talked about. I'm sure it was all about crayon colors and our favorite letters of the alphabet; after all, we were first graders, for goodness' sakes.

Mark Peterson and I became friends and would often play together in our neighborhood. Our moms became friends, too. Mom remembers one day while Mark and I were wrestling in the yard, she and Mark's mom sat and watched through the window. I was very big for my age and Mark was very small. Mark's mom turned to mine and said, *"You can tell that Sean is doing his best not to hurt him."*

Whatever emotion or circumstance I was experiencing, it was always made better when I could retreat to my comfort zone, the living room of our little apartment, with food. Did it start as early as four? Yes, it did, and continued as I became an adult, husband, and father (not necessarily in that order*).*

In a world where my comfort zone was often shattered and my fears reluctantly faced, food was good. It tasted good, incredible really, and while I enjoyed the peaceful moments and flavors of whatever I was eating, everything was right with the world. Another emotional eater, a *food addict* was born. The positive experience of that comfort became addicting. As negative circumstances would arise, brought on, invited really, by my peaceful, friendly personality, and refusal to stand up for myself, I would run faster, back to the place where I knew everything was good.

It was a vicious cycle of pain and comfort, where the comfort inadvertently led to more pain, and the pain required more and more comfort. I was lucky to be so young and living in a wonderfully sheltered environment of our little apartment, not knowing what drugs and alcohol were, good thing. My comfort, my shelter, my vicious cycle swirled around food. The result was childhood obesity, at a time when those words were rarely put together, in a time when I was most usually the only overweight kid in class.

Mom dated every now and then and I wasn't a fan of anyone she chose. There wasn't a man good enough for my mother. I felt like my perfectly sheltered environment was somehow threatened. I was completely dependent on Mom, and any attention she gave anyone else, especially a fella named Wayne, just upset me. I didn't like Wayne and she knew it.

Wayne tried his best to make me like him. He even used food. He was good. *How did he know I loved biscuits and gravy?* He woke me up one morning and asked if I would go to the store with him to pick up ingredients to prepare homemade biscuits and sausage gravy. Maybe there was hope for this guy after all. Our relationship didn't have time to develop, because as soon as Mom became pregnant, Wayne came around less and less. My suspicions were right, he wasn't good enough for my mother. And now Mom didn't have time or energy to date, my little brother Shane was coming soon, and he was going to be a welcomed addition to our little apartment.

"Will he ever stop crying?" My goodness, babies are loud. *"Can we take him back?"* It was a half serious question. I wasn't adjusting very smoothly to the idea of sharing Mom's attention. But the more I got to know him, the more I loved and understood my role as big

brother. Shane was very special. At five years old, I had no idea how much he would eventually teach me about love and compassion.

Shane was born with what the doctors referred to as "mild mental retardation." I hate the word "retarded." Shane was *mentally challenged* and in a lot of ways showed signs of being autistic, although he was never officially diagnosed with autism. I knew that part of my job would be to protect him. The idea kind of made me nervous because I wasn't sure about protecting me. I knew being different attracted unwanted attention, and Shane was different. I needed to be a strong big brother because who knew what was coming? The unknown answer to that question gave me a wafer-thin strength that left me emotionally fragile most of the time.

Somewhere around eight years old, I was walking home from school, finished being the fat kid for the day and headed toward an after-school snack within the safe confines of F-207. There was a group of older boys, probably late teens, maybe early twenties, hanging out by a vehicle close to the staircase that led to our front door. I was almost home free. As I approached, their attention turned to me. One of them started laughing as he said the words that would embed in my brain forever. It didn't mean anything to those guys, it was just one of many laughs in their day-to-day lives, but to me, it cut deep and gave me a complex that has plagued me my entire life. He said, *"Hey, you need to wear a bra."* It hurt bad, those words. They hit me harder than any bullying or remarks about my weight up to that moment in time. I made it up the stairs before letting the tears flow, and as the tears dried, I was changed underneath. I would never swim again without a shirt on, I would never change shirts in front of anyone, I would always carry their careless words on the edge of my brain, ready to come front and center if my new boundary was ever threatened, and it was many times.

"Anderson, skins!" shouted Mr. Hayes across the gymnasium. It was third and fourth grade basketball practice. I wasn't the athletic type, but when you're attending a really small school like Pleasant View, everybody must play, or you can't put a team on the court. Even

me, the heaviest kid in school, was allowed to suit up and play. *"Anderson, get that shirt off and get in there."* He wasn't stopping. He knew how I was, he knew I was self-conscious about my chest, he didn't care. *Why was tall and slim Tommy on the shirts side? What about Matt?* Matt was on the shirts team, too. I wanted to be on the shirts practice team *permanently*. If asked why he pressed, Mr. Hayes would have probably said he was just trying to get me to face and break free from this silly little hang-up. But it wasn't silly to me. It was very serious. And if Mr. Hayes didn't realize how serious it was at the moment, he certainly did several moments later.

I wasn't facing my insecurities that day. I quietly turned around and walked toward the door. I didn't look back one time, I was done for the day and season. I was only a three-minute walk from the comfort of something good to eat in the safe confines of our little apartment. I didn't care about the team, or Mr. Hayes, or anything other than protecting myself from the torment I was certain to face if I exposed my fatty boy boobs.

Chapter Two

Wearing the Target

My weight wasn't the only thing that made me stand out. I was a fat, scared of my own shadow white kid, the awkward duck in a neighborhood that was roughly eighty percent African American. Being the fat kid was just a bonus, so to speak, another way for me to be noticeably different in a community where everyone struggled to survive and most everyone seemed to be looking for something, anything to distract them from the reality that surrounded. Many times, they found me.

Edwin was a slender black kid, nearly half a foot shorter than me. Physically, I shouldn't have been intimidated by him, but mentally, he had my number, and he took full advantage of the power I allowed. And he wasn't the only one.

Frankie was also smaller than me. Wait a second, everyone my age was smaller than me. Anyway, for Frankie, our difference in size was the *only reason* he needed for me to become a target. Frankie, a Native American, had long black hair and killer looks. I don't mean he was good looking, he just looked like he could kill you and not even give it a second thought. At least, that's what I told myself. Maybe he was a real pussy cat deep down, who knows. But I doubt it. I trembled with fear every time he decided to make issue with me. Whatever he really was didn't matter. To me, he was terrifying.

Getting made fun of was a daily experience in those early years, and sadly, often times I would play along. If I smiled or laughed outwardly, maybe they would decide to stop, or so I thought. If I held the pain and tears inside while at school, I could let the tears go as soon as I made it to my room. But the hurt feelings, the lonely, desperate emotions, those were just building. And when the fat jokes turned into bullying, the feelings transformed from hurt to painful terror.

Edwin and Frankie bullied me all the time. Never together, always on their own, but with similar dynamics. They loved to watch me squirm as they controlled me in every way. *Why did I give them that power?* Because the idea of fighting back was scarier than what they were doing to me. If I fought back, I thought, there's a chance I could be on the losing end of a fight, and failing in a fist fight situation, in my mind, was potentially *deadly.* And so I allowed it to continue, always wondering, *why me?* Out of all the other kids in school and around the neighborhood, why am I *the one?* I was the fat kid, I was an easy target with a proven track record of never standing up for myself, that's why.

The dynamics may have been similar, but Edwin and Frankie had very different styles of bullying. Edwin would often resort to extortion in exchange for "protection" from him. Frankie wanted to beat me up, simply "because you're the biggest kid in school." He actually told me that one time. I'll never forget the time Frankie showed up at our apartment and ordered me outside for a beat down. I stood at the door, on the safe side of the threshold, and told him that I was grounded. Mom didn't have a single clue what was really going on, so she corrected me, *"Sean, you're not grounded, you go on out and play with your friends."* I wasn't ready to tell Mom what was really happening, so I nervously shuffled outside and immediately started begging for my life to be spared.

"Frankie, please don't hit me. What did I do to you? Let's be friends, okay? I don't want to fight, I don't even know how to fight, so really, I wouldn't be much of a challenge." Frankie looked at me with a steely glare and then, *"How much money you got?" "Uh, like two bucks." "Go get it and I'll leave you alone."* Giving Frankie two-weeks worth of my allowance was better than getting hit, and considering Edwin's rates, it was a real bargain.

11

Edwin would threaten to beat me up unless I brought him a steady supply of Coke-a-Cola six packs. The kid loved soda apparently, maybe he wasn't allowed to drink it at home, I don't know. I *almost never* said no to Edwin. If I couldn't "pay" him, I would often beg for more time to satisfy his demands. It was like dealing with a fifth-grade mafia boss. My poor mother, I would tell her that we were having another party at school, and that I had volunteered to bring the soda. Even when we couldn't afford it, I knew that Mom would get the money to buy whatever I needed, somehow, some way, even if it meant borrowing the money from Grandma and Grandpa. She didn't know the real reason I was taking the six-packs of Coke to school, I was afraid to tell her, not because of what she might do, but because of the retaliation I might face for telling. *Okay, honestly, it was also in fear of what she might do.* Regardless, I knew that eventually I had to let her in on my torment.

I started missing school on a regular basis. I never skipped; I was just always sick and needed to stay home. Mom would take me to the doctor and they wouldn't find anything wrong with me, except one time—they found a stomach ulcer. A nine-year-old with an ulcer—from stress, no doubt. I remember being happy that the doctor actually found something. *See, I wasn't always faking!* Dr. Wright, my pediatrician, once leaned over my emergency room triage bed and asked, *"Sean, do you have cable TV at home?"* He was trying to figure out why I seemed so happy to be undergoing barium enemas and numerous other invasive tests in search of my "sickness." Anything was better than going to school and facing Edwin or Frankie.

Eventually, the school started cracking down, even showing up at our apartment and demanding my attendance. I pushed the absence policy to the limit every school year and it wasn't long before I started to realize, I had to "go public" with the bullying. I had to tell my mom and the school why I hated going to school so badly. This wasn't going to be easy, but necessary.

As soon as I told Mom what was going on, she was ready to unleash a response that would surely label her the craziest mom in the apartment complex and I would be forever known as the biggest momma's boy on the planet. I was and proudly am a momma's boy, but at that age I didn't need anything else to stock the ammunition piles of my aggressors. Mom's response, even though I had to talk her down from a history making stand, made me feel safe. Mom was on my side, it was going to be alright. She was gritting her teeth mad, and when Momma starts talking through gritted teeth, somebody better watch out. We decided that a trip to the principal, Mr. McEwen, was in order first thing the next morning.

As Mom and I approached the principal's office, Edwin made eye contact with me, he wasn't speaking, just glaring, something he did so well. His glaring always left me to create my own story about what he was thinking and how he was going to kill me. He had to know that something was up, because this wasn't a normal start to a typical school day. Mr. McEwen had perfectly groomed short, straight black hair and a neatly trimmed black mustache. He was a major authority figure in my life, the one that would personally show up at my apartment door demanding my attendance and wondering why going to school was such a major issue for me. He was about to find out.

Through nervous tears, in the presence of a loving and very protective mother who was doing her best not to interject commentary along the way, I spilled the details of my constant torment. Mr. McEwen listened intently and came up with a solution in one simple six-word question. *"Why don't you just hit him?"*

This wasn't what I wanted to hear. I wanted to hear how I would be assigned a personal body guard or maybe put into some kind of special isolated learning environment. *Why didn't I just hit him? What kind of question was that coming from a principal?* Mr. McEwen was getting straight to the heart of the matter, with a solution that would have worked with Edwin and quite possibly changed the course of my childhood, but wow, oh my...*I had to answer him now, oh boy, here we go . . .*

"I don't want to get suspended from school." That was it, that was my reason, or at least the one I gave Mr. McEwen. I skipped right over the real answer, how I was deathly afraid to fight, in fear of becoming helplessly pummeled by the feet and fist of my attacker. I must have forgotten who I was talking to, Mr. McEwen *was* the principal; if anyone is suspended, he's the one that makes that ultimate decision. And he quickly let me know that my fear wasn't necessary. At least the fear I falsely expressed, after all. I would have *loved* being suspended, at least then I could stay home without the principal showing up on my doorstep.

He offered, *"Sean, the next time Edwin threatens you, you haul off and punch him as hard as you can in the face, and I will look the other way." Now what?* He just challenged me to stand up for myself, and until that plan goes horribly wrong, we didn't have anymore reason to be in his office. I was extremely dissatisfied with this solution, the primal quality to fight just wasn't in me, there had to be a peaceful solution. *Maybe I could offer Edwin the new plastic two-liter bottles instead of cans.* Mr. McEwen knew what I didn't realize at the time: You can't negotiate with a terrorist, even when the terrorist is a fifth-grade bully.

Mom wasn't necessarily satisfied with Mr. McEwen's solution either. Maybe she understood that violence might have ended my bully-victim relationship with Edwin, but would do little to really change the underlying psychology that made Edwin a fantastic bully and me a wonderful victim. Besides, Mom knew I wasn't a fighter and the thought of someone trying to physically harm me left her scrambling for a better solution.

That's when she decided to do something courageous. It was something that I wasn't comfortable with at all, but her mind was made up. She was going behind enemy lines, into the very nest that had nurtured the bully that was Edwin. She was headed down the sidewalk that led from our place to Edwin's apartment. Mom was ready to have a big talk with Edwin's mother. In my eyes, it was one of the bravest things I had ever witnessed.

What if she gets ambushed? What if Edwin's mom turns out to be an older version of Edwin? I guess if Mom emerges from their apartment and we start delivering groceries to their doorstep, I'll know. Mom wasn't showing any signs of fear. Mom asked if I wanted to go, too, but I don't think I could have handled being *in there.* Shane and I watched from our living room perch, faces pressed against the glass, as Mom bravely marched into enemy territory. She knocked and Edwin's mom answered the door, inviting her inside. *She was inside Edwin's apartment!*

I had to stop and pray for her safety at that moment, *this was intense. Please, Lord, protect my Momma from the dangers that surely surrounds her in this moment.*

The seconds seemed like minutes and the minutes seemed like hours. *What were they possibly talking about this long?* My prayers for her safety were answered as she emerged from the other side, without a scratch, and slowly made her way back up the sidewalk to our peaceful little place. *Was that a smile on the face of Edwin's mom? How strange, she smiles?*

"She said that you need to hit him," Mom said with a heavy-exhausted sigh. *Hit him? His own mother said to hit him?*

I couldn't believe my ears. It turns out that Edwin's mom knew another side of Edwin that was completely unimaginable to me, she knew *the real Edwin.* Her solution was the same as Mr. McEwen's. She didn't care that her son might get hurt, rather, she was hoping he might learn a lesson. I needed to learn a lesson, too, about standing up for myself, but the fear, *oh dear,* the fear was just so paralyzing.

Mom knew that it didn't matter how many endorsements of violence I had or from whom they came, there wasn't any way I would ever throw that potentially life-changing punch. It wasn't in me to throw. The life changes I needed couldn't be helped with my fist. We had to deal with the issues that made me different, the issues that

15

attracted the bullying in the first place. I needed a diet and some counseling. Appointments were made and we felt good about it all.

I've always been an optimist. I can remember walking to school in complete dread of what I might face, but comforting myself with this thought: *At a little after three PM, no matter what happens today, I'll be safe and sound in front of the TV, eating an after-school snack in the safe confines of our little home.* It was my "internal hope mechanism," my instinct of survival, knowing that I would somehow make it back to that comfortable place, no matter what transpired at school.

The therapist recognized my optimism and internal hope right away. In fact, my counseling sessions ended after the first visit, when the counselor told my mom, *"There's nothing wrong with Sean, he's a survivor, he's going to be okay."* I'm a survivor? Wow, *that's pretty cool,* I thought. *What does that mean? Was it some kind of superhero power?* Or did it mean I would find a way to cope with whatever was pressing, finding a way back to our apartment and that after-school snack, despite everything. *What about that diet?*

Doctor Wright was my pediatrician and I was always giving him challenges. Whatever pretend symptoms I needed to get out of school, he had to try to figure out what they really were and how to treat them. Dr. Wright was a very smart man, and when he asked me about our TV channels at home, he was letting me know that he knew the truth. There wasn't anything medically urgent that needed attention, other than my weight. And for that, he had a wonderful solution. He handed Mom a one-thousand calorie diet, complete with menus, and ordered her to put me "on it."

There it was in black and white, the solution to all of my problems. If I would eat exactly what was on that list, in that order and quantity, I would magically become thin and all of my childhood troubles would dissolve into thin air. This was the answer. It's funny, because even at that young age, I knew that it wasn't a realistic solution. *Poached eggs?* I'd never even heard of such a thing and now I'm supposed to eat them?

When we realized that the practicality of this thousand-calorie diet wasn't fitting for our lifestyle, we started looking at other weight loss solutions. Slender Bars, Figurines, and Aids were all given a shot. Remember Aids? They resembled caramels, in fact, I think they were caramels with a different name and an inferior recipe. When you would experience hunger, simply eat a few of these little candies, and you would make it until your next meal. *Brilliant!* Or so it seemed. They were a little too tasty, a little too much like candy, and a little too easy. I ate them like candy and they never stopped me from eating more at mealtime *or any other time.* And the name, oh my, *Aids* quickly disappeared or perhaps was renamed, sometime in the early eighties when a horrible new disease was discovered.

The Slender Bars and Figurine Bars were simply candy bars to me. You know what was good? Put the Figurine bars in the freezer, let 'em get nice and cold, then enjoy! They were supposed to be a meal-replacement diet plan, designed to drop the pounds. Instead, they were just another wonderful snack, ate up by what was quickly becoming an all-out food addiction.

We even tried packing a lunch at home, even though my school lunch was free, but that didn't set well with me. *You mean I have to eat this turkey-ham sandwich on super thin "diet" bread and carrot sticks while everyone else enjoys the amazingly delicious school lunch?* The "take my own lunch" idea didn't last long, and we tried it several different times. I wanted to eat what everyone else was eating. Everyone else but Scott Henderson, he always brought his lunch from home, and for reasons I didn't understand, he actually preferred it that way, or so it seemed. All I know is, Scott never had a weight problem and didn't seem to be the least bit phased on cinnamon roll and pizza day or chocolate milk Friday.

I looked forward to lunchtime at school. The entire school would fill with the smell of whatever was on the menu that day, and we would often try and guess what it was by the amazing smell wafting through the halls, or maybe it was just me who did that. The best day was always cinnamon roll and pizza day. I would often scan the lunch trays of the other kids, just to see what they didn't care to eat. If it was Friday fish day, then . . . *"You want your hushpuppies? Can I have them?"* My cousin Steve and I had a contest one time, with the goal being to see who could accumulate the most hushpuppies. I ended with over a hundred of the tasty things, eating not even half, but still enough to make me feel sick. *It was hushpuppy heaven.* I wasn't eating for comfort that day; I was eating for fun. But really, my addiction to food wasn't just about emotional comfort. Food was everything. It's what I turned to when I was sad, happy, when I was bored, or when I was trying to set some kind of school hushpuppy eating record.

Perhaps diets and counseling weren't the answer for me. Maybe I just needed sports and a positive male influence. In hindsight, I really should have shared with the counselor how much the absence of my father bothered me. It was an issue that I simply wasn't emotionally equipped to handle and I didn't want to acknowledge, unless forced to explain, like the time the school had a father-son basketball game.

"Where's your dad, Sean?" Timmy Mutz had a dad at home, a cool dad with a motorcycle. From Timmy's perspective, everyone had a dad. Where was mine he asked? *"Uh, he, uh, was killed in Vietnam."* It was a lie, of course, in fact it was totally opposite of the truth I would later discover. My biological father bravely and honorably survived two tours in Vietnam, the second tour in an effort to keep his brother states-side and safe. What an amazing thing to do for your little brother. That's the kind of love I had for Shane, it made perfect sense.

Veyon Haynes made it home from the jungles of Vietnam just in time to meet my mom and help create me. For reasons I didn't know or understand, and my dad probably didn't understand at the time, he had to retreat from the responsibility of being my father. Perhaps the war left his mental and emotional capacity at its limit, having nothing left for me or my mother. I didn't know and it didn't matter.

Saying he was dead was far easier than trying to answer the flood of unanswerable questions that might come if I had told the truth. *"He died,"* kind of killed that conversation. *How did he die?* The war, of course, shot and killed. *"Nobody knows the details of the battle that killed him, it's top secret."* I told this sensational lie so many times, I almost started believing it was true. Saying it was "top secret," made me feel important. Like, *Hey, my dad was special, so there.* Call it a son's love, or whatever, I had never known him, never seen or touched him, yet I took pride in his wartime bravery. I was proud to be a son of a brave soldier. My dad wasn't really dead as far as I knew, but I was still several years from actually confirming his existence. I knew the war didn't physically kill him, or I would have never been born.

Every obstacle we faced, the neighborhood we called home, the poverty, the bullying, my childhood obesity, all of it, was because my dad wasn't there for us. *That's what I told myself.* Like his presence would have magically transformed our existence into some kind of great American dream family. It wasn't true, in fact, I'm almost certain, given his condition upon returning from war, our lives could have been much worse had he stuck around. One of his greatest gifts was his absence from my childhood.

By the summer of 1981, I was busy playing ten and under baseball. I was the worst player in the history of Stillwater Parks and Recreation. I was the fat kid that refused to tuck my shirt into my baseball pants. I never once hit the ball in ten and under play. The only time I got on base was when I had a "good eye, good eye" and drew a walk. Otherwise, I was the strikeout king of the little league.

Despite my horrible play, my status was bumped up to semi-cool kid one warm summer night when a motorcycle came rumbling up to the baseball game. The guy on the bike was there to see me play. And he really didn't care if I hit the ball or not, *good thing,* because I wasn't hitting that ball, *ever.* His name was Clarke Hodson, a bearded young man, a college student assigned to me by the Big Brothers Big Sisters Program.

He watched me play, cheering me on, and then, in what was quite possibly the coolest thing ever, he offered to give me a ride home on his motorcycle. I looked at Mom with my big, blue "please let me" eyes, and she agreed to meet us back at the apartment. As I climbed onto the back of that *hog*, okay, actually, I think it was a Honda, all of the other kids looked at me with envy, or at least, that's what I told myself they were doing. Yep, he was my big brother, and his positive influence on me was wonderful, but it didn't stop my developing relationship with food. And neither did being the worst little league baseball player in the history of the game. I will say this, as I rode home on the back of that giant Honda machine, food was the furthest thing from my mind.

Clarke came along at a crucial time in my childhood. I needed that one-on-one interaction with a positive male role model, something I didn't have at home. I looked up to my grandpa and Uncle Keith, but my relationship with Clarke was different. Class was in session whenever we were together. If we were headed to the science museum in Oklahoma City, you could bet I was answering complicated math problems all the way there, and I loved it.

I loved the attention, I loved the escape from reality that our weekly hang-out time provided. Clarke made me feel important, he made me feel smart, he gave me some confidence, and he always did his best to set an amazing example. Clarke was athletic, too, and he even had a volleyball court in his backyard. I think about his influence and what it was to me and what it could have been had I not been so emotionally starved for positive male interaction. Instead of learning about physical fitness and learning how to love learning, two things that surely would have righted my childhood deficiencies, I was constantly cherishing, becoming addicted really to his attention. I separated my life away from Clarke from my time with him, he was an escape, cherished moments of nurturing, and when our visit was finished for the day, I'd reluctantly go back into the same existence as before, but always looking forward to our next adventure.

Clarke took me out and showed me how to do things. I'll never forget the time he told me to get behind the wheel of his truck. He taught me how to drive at eleven years old, because if anything happened to him while he cut firewood with a chainsaw, then I needed to be able to drive him to a hospital. I could have done it. While I was with him, I could do anything. He showed me compassion, he showed me tenderness, he showed me integrity, and he taught me that those things were cool, even coming from a man. Clarke was the real deal. But as his love and attention grew toward his college sweetheart and his studies, we had less and less time together, and eventually the day came when our time was done. I loved Clarke and our time together, I did, and it was nothing less than pure heartbreak when the time came for us to move forward apart. I remember laying in bed and crying my eyes out, I was emotionally broken. But looking back now, I realize that my obsession over his attention and my closeness to him, became too much. Too much for me to really learn anything that I could put into practice in my little boy life. I was too busy focusing on the escape he provided me, not allowing his influence to soak into practical use at the time. Although his influence on me, I have no doubt, did its part in making me a better father to my daughters.

The second big brother assigned to me didn't have a chance. Clarke set the bar too high. When the guy (I don't even remember his name) took me to his parents' farm, I couldn't have been less interested. To me, it was an afternoon of dodging hot steamy piles of manure. I guess it's all about perspective. I may have attended a small independent school on the outskirts of town, but I was a city boy. Maybe the look on my twelve-year-old face gave it away because somehow we both knew that our time together was limited to one visit. I remember him telling me about the virtues of a hard days' work on the farm, and how it would keep me in shape. I guess he felt the need to be educational, offering something that might help me lose weight. Maybe he was thinking about giving me a summer job or something, I don't know. I wasn't really paying attention because I was too busy missing Clarke, missing the comfort of our apartment, and wondering where to find the window seal holding the freshly baked and cooling apple pie. *This is a farm house in the middle of Oklahoma, surely someone has baked a pie here today. Can we go to McDonald's?*

Despite our circumstances with poverty, not having my father in our lives, the bullying, the constant struggle with weight issues and me never wanting to go to school, I was a pretty happy kid.

Maybe it was that *internal hope mechanism* thingy, or the *survivor* title given me by the therapist, whatever it was, I was a lucky kid, blessed always and I knew it. Whatever made me sad, food and my momma's embrace would make it better. My line of least resistance was developing at a very young age and it came complete with an all-you-can-eat buffet.

There were times when my larger size made me the hero. Long before William "The Refrigerator" Perry came along, I was known in the neighborhood as "The Tank." The green yards in front of the apartment buildings were perfect for tackle football games. The grass was soft and gentle, with concrete sidewalks leading up to apartment doors and serving as yardage markers. As long as you didn't get tackled on the sidewalk, you were going to be alright. I'm not sure who had the bright idea to let me be a ball carrier, but whoever it was, was way ahead of Mike Ditka. My job was simple: Take the hand-off and run through everyone. My size made it easier to blast through piles of smaller kids, and if they were hanging on to me, I could drag them a few more feet, just enough to get me away from the sidewalk before I crashed to the ground under three or four tacklers. I was "The Tank," and everyone wanted me on their team for a little while, until my weight gain slowed me down a little too much, or maybe we just stopped playing football in the yard, or maybe I just stopped playing.

As I try to understand the elements that came together, making me a morbidly obese young man, I don't see any of the elements that have contributed to the modern-day childhood obesity epidemic. We didn't have computers. Cartoons were something you watched on Saturday mornings. And until my early teens, we didn't have video games, although I did have a Pong-like knock-off game, but it was never enough to hold my attention for very long. If you wanted to play a video game, you actually had to walk down to the arcade with some quarters. I can remember my cousin Steve and me walking and sometimes riding our bikes, over a mile with a single quarter between us. We were after the Galaga game at the Humpty Dumpty grocery store. We took turns playing, with each of us playing at least two turns, as long as we made it to the first bonus level to get that extra spaceship. It didn't take much to entertain us. The answer wasn't in our activities; it was in our inactivities, in our behaviors around food. That's where the difference was found. My dependency was on food and the comfort and goodness it provided. Other kids my age might have put their emotional energy into non-food related escapes, but I didn't understand those kids at all. *I was different.*

I kept my food behaviors under wraps and in private, most of the time, but sometimes my food lusting compulsions would come out. Aunt Connie, my cousin Steve's mom, had a keen eye for my habits. I'll never forget the time we were all at a family get-together and I found myself alone with a beautiful uncut cake. Aunt Connie was the cake baker in the family, and this one-of-a-kind creation from her came complete with pecan halves on top. It was a work of art and I couldn't get my mind off of how good it must have tasted. I guess I realized that someone might notice if a piece was cut early, but for some reason, I didn't think anyone would notice if the pecans were missing. I stood right there in the kitchen of my great grandma and grandpa Hadley's eyeing that cake, wanting it, craving it, needing just a little. While everyone else was in the living room playing and listening to music, or visiting, and the other kids were outside running and playing, I quietly picked off and ate every single pecan from the top of that cake. I knew it was wrong, because I was in a hurry to get the job done. My rushed pecan devouring must have left some icing on my lips—a dead giveaway, but I didn't notice—I was too happy and full. After Aunt Connie walked in and discovered the mutilated cake, it took her all of about three seconds to figure out who was responsible. She shouted, *"Seanboy, what's wrong with you?"* She was not happy. And as far as I was concerned, nothing was *wrong with me*. I just really loved pecans . . . especially with icing, on top of a cake, *didn't everybody?*

As my early childhood came to a close and the young teen in me started thinking about girls, I knew something had to change. Before I could start working on losing weight, I had to deal with Edwin again. It was the first day of junior high school. All of us Pleasant View kids were taken out of the country and the projects and put into the Stillwater School system, complete with lockers and changing classes every hour. This was a different world, but it didn't take long before Edwin showed up to remind me that some things never change. *But they had to change.*

Edwin walked up to me that day and glared at me while he started the old familiar harassment from all of the years before. I never hit Edwin like Mr. McEwen and Edwin's own mother suggested and encouraged. But what I did on that day was different than any response I'd ever given Edwin before.

Remember I said earlier, that *I almost never said no* to Edwin? That first day of junior high would be the exception to the rule. I turned around and gave Edwin a look so serious, that he was speechless. It was my turn to say something. And right there, in the halls of Stillwater Junior High School, as I paused from trying to figure out the combination lock for my bright yellow locker, I stood up for myself.

I didn't throw a punch. I simply said, in a very slow, dramatic tone, *"Edwin, it's not going to work here."* Edwin looked confused and believe it or not, a little nervous. I was always the one left wondering how he was going to kill me, trying to figure out his twisted bully-minded ways, and now—I left him wondering what "it's not going to work here," meant. I didn't really know myself, all I knew was, with the emotions and nervousness that I carried into that first day of Junior High, the last thing I needed was Edwin's terror and dread. And Edwin obviously didn't want to find out, calling my bluff was just too risky, so he walked away, and he never bullied me again. It turned a page for me, a new chapter—a new perspective. I wanted everyone to like me, and if I could find a girl to really like me, that would be awesome, too.

By the way, Edwin and Frankie both ended up in prison as adults, the same prison in fact. I would often joke about someday visiting them and how fun that might be, but I'll never make that trip. It did make for some funny stand-up comedy material, how I would tell them that I was just dropping in on my way to my new job on the pardon and parole board. I even talked about taking Edwin a six pack of Coke cans, but not being able to fit it through the little holes in the plexiglass that divided the prisoners from the visitors. I actually entertained this trip idea until an anonymous blog reader made me think about something very important concerning Edwin and Frankie, and my desire to see them behind bars. *We were just kids.* And if my emotional and psychological deficiencies led me to food addiction and childhood obesity, theirs led them to bullying and a troubled life. We all ended up imprisoned by the consequences of our choices. Mine was metaphorically, imprisoned by obesity, theirs literally, imprisoned by the justice system. Revengeful pleasure in their suffering has no place in real forgiveness. And our childhood transgressions must be forgiven. Although, I'm not sure Aunt Connie would trust me to this day, around one of her pecan-topped custom cakes.

Chapter Three

Tears of a Clown

The start of junior high was also the start of a new awareness within me. I could see it all around me, young junior high love blossoming. Never before did I feel so invisible. By the time I turned thirteen, I was approaching one hundred pounds overweight, and the girls were not looking my way, unless it was to make some kind of disgusted face or because I said something or did something funny, often at my expense. Anything to get their attention, right? The guys that attracted all of the crush-laden attention were the jocks. Mike Van Pelt, Chris Holt, Rob Lorenzo, you know, guys with really cool names. The cooler the name, the more attractive they seemed to the girls in our school. *Sean Anderson* wasn't the coolest name in the world. *How could I compete with a Mike Van Pelt or a Rob Lorenzo?* You couldn't find movie stars with better names. But there they were, ruling the halls and claiming the attention of every female around. I often thought, if these girls would only take the time to know me, you know, look past my physical appearance, they would find an amazing heart. They would discover that the greatest guy in the school was hiding behind a hundred pounds of fat and serious insecurities. Despite the insecurities and image I projected, I knew deep down who I was and what they were missing out on.

Maybe I just needed to let my feelings be known, you know, take a chance and speak up. I remember in eighth grade, deciding to do just that . . . speak up. The object of my eighth-grade affection wasn't the tallest, or the blondest, or the head cheerleader, or the most popular girl in school, but she was everything to me, she was perfection, and she didn't even know. The idea of being dropped off at Cowboy Mall and just hanging out with her, talking, *and uh, maybe we could play some video games, or I could buy her some frozen yogurt,* would have been a dream come true.

If I could just show her my awesome Pac-Man skills, she would forever be impressed, after all, I had the pattern memorized. Seriously, all the way to the eighth key, you know, when even eating the big power dot fails to turn them blue, yeah—one quarter would last me an hour. Isn't it fitting that my favorite game was all about eating everything in sight as fast as you can while trying to dodge an early death? But, anyway, this isn't a story about Pac-Man.

Fourth hour would be the time, English class, it was on. I was so nervous all day, leading up to the moment I asked her "out." I entered class that day, making eye contact with her right away. I smiled, and she didn't, but that was normal. I'll just keep smiling.

Looking back on it, it must have came off kind of creepy, this fixed smile of mine. I was trying to let her know that I came in peace, that I was friendly and nice. My desk was right across the aisle from her, she slightly ahead of me in her row. Class was almost over when I finally found the nerve to lean forward and whisper my sweet desire. *"Would you go out with me?"* Big smile, Sean, *show her those teeth, very nice.* What happened next was seriously over the top in the rejection department. A simple, *"I'm sorry, I can't, but thank you, anyway,"* would have been perfect.

Instead, her face contorted like someone had shoved a teaspoon of turpentine in her mouth, followed by, *"Ewwwww! I would never go out with you, gross!" Gross,* really? Why such a long *"ewwwww"* anyway? *Was I really that repulsive? Was this shirt showing my boy boobs a little too much, or what?* All that smiling for nothing? *I just wanted to make her smile.*

My obesity made me different, pure and simple. And the social consequences of my differences had now changed. The differences in the younger me created a personality that attracted the bullies, and now, the differences in me no longer attracted the bullies, but repelled the girls. In my mind, the only thing that separated me from total teenage happiness was being fat.

I wasn't getting picked on anymore and the girls didn't like me *in that way* because I was fat. So, I lose the weight, I get the girl, no more bullying, teenage romance, and we all live happily ever after.

What if I became interested in sports? *Yeah, that's it.* I had a revelation. Sports was the answer. Never mind that I was the worst little league baseball player in the history of the game, never mind that I was the slowest runner in the entire school—no, no—check that, in the entire region. At Pleasant View, everybody ran track, it was part of P.E. class, even me. So, somewhere in this world exist old track meet records that prove I was the slowest runner in an eight-county region. *One-hundred-yard dash? You mean, all at once without stopping?*

About the time I decided that I would lose this weight and become a super athlete who never got bullied and always had a date, my size started getting attention from the coaches around school. Perfect timing, huh?

They didn't see this pathetic fat kid, oh no—they saw potential. They could see a young man who was already six foot tall, never mind the extra one hundred pounds of fat, they could run that off of me. Mr. McClain was the first to pull me aside. He called me into his office to verbalize this attention. I'll never forget that day. It was like a crossroads for me. A choice was going to be made with two very different consequences. Mr. McClain was hyping me up like a division one college football recruiter. *He was good.*

At first, I had no idea why Mr. McClain was calling me into his office that day. But the more he talked, the better I felt about myself.

"Sean, you are a big boy," he said, *"And if you let us get you into that weight room every day, and you lift weights and workout with the wrestlers, you could be a powerhouse in high school football."* I told you he was good.

Let him take you and mold you into exactly what you dream of being, I said to myself, before he interrupted with, *"You be in the weight room tomorrow after school, and we'll get you started."* Well, I wasn't in trouble, that was good. I was being recruited, kind of, and it was exactly what I wanted, I thought. But it also scared me because, well—if they make me take my shirt off, I'm walking. I did it in fourth grade basketball and I'll do it again. And then there's the little problem with my right arm strength.

My right arm is shorter than my left and it's considerably weaker. The bones are not positioned correctly in my right arm because I was born with a broken arm. The problem was, this little broken baby arm wasn't identified at birth. The doctor told my mom that my muscles were under-developed and that she needed to work out my little arm every day, and hopefully someday I would move it on my own. My baby bones eventually hardened enough, despite the daily doctor-ordered workout, for me to move my right arm on my own, but they fused together incorrectly, forever affecting my athletic capabilities. I knew this. This was why I couldn't throw a ball very hard in little league. This is why lifting weights made me nervous because you can't balance a bar when one arm is dramatically weaker than the other. Showing up in that weight room as Mr. McClain suggested, meant facing all of this, and dealing directly with the possible teasing it might attract.

I avoided everything that might attract teasing. Everything except having a horrendous emotional dependency on food—that was my catch twenty-two. Mr. McClain was offering me a way out, he and the other coaches would have helped me, but I couldn't get over my insane defenses of my insecurities, even though I knew that their help could possibly change my life for the better. A crossroads, absolutely . . . it was.

The next day, after school, I was at McDonald's eating instead of in the weight room lifting. A big choice was made. And the consequences of that choice would dramatically affect me the rest of my adolescent years.

I avoided Mr. McClain like the plague for a very long time. He never once called me back into his office. He knew that a decision was made and it didn't involve his vision of my future as a top high school college football prospect. I was wrapped up in myself really tight. Deep down, I dreamed of being free from all of the restrictions my obesity created, either real or imagined, but I was too dependent on the food for comfort. Often times, the comfort was sought, in refuge from the restrictions created by being fat. It's that vicious cycle I was talking about earlier. I was quickly discovering a comfort zone and acceptance of what it meant, or what I could be, and still be excessively overweight.

I could still be the class clown, and make everyone laugh. I mean, really, *isn't that what I ultimately wanted?* Everyone to like me? And maybe I could find a sport that I could do well, despite my size and mild physical deformity. I started getting more and more interested in Mrs. Mason's speech and drama class—there was an upcoming school play, maybe I could audition for a role!

And what about sports? *How about Putt-Putt?* Don't laugh, it's a sport. In fact, in the early to mid-eighties, ESPN would televise the Professional Putters Putt-Putt Championships. *This was it,* these two elements would absolutely change my life for the better! I would become the school actor, comedian, and Putt-Putt champion, yeah—that would fix me.

I wasn't going to change my behaviors with food that were just making me fatter, so my life and activities would just need to adapt and accept me . . . *the funny fat kid with a deadly stroke ten feet from the hole, from behind the triangle block, and banked off the bumper board.* I could Putt-Putt like nobody's business, *or at least that's how I like to remember it all.*

Watching the Tonight Show with Johnny Carson was a regular habit at our little apartment. I had the pleasure of witnessing Louie Anderson's very first appearance. *Check that out,* I thought, *everybody loves him, and he's fat, but he's funny.* And what made him funny? He spent a good deal of his short set, making fun of himself. I'm not saying Louie taught me the fundamentals of self-deprecating humor, I'm just saying it was a perfect example of someone else doing exactly what I already had discovered.

I wasn't alone or abnormal, but in a way, I had become the bullied and the bully, all rolled up in one. If it made everyone smile, and even better, laugh, then I would absolutely do it again and again. Like a politician, I would try to win everyone over, one laugh at a time. Or, I could find a bigger stage and get everyone all at once. The school play was coming up—and it was decided. I was auditioning.

"The Happiness Machine," was the title of our school play, about a machine in a department store that automatically tells if two people are compatible. Or was it, *"The Perfect Couple,"* doesn't matter. Whatever the title, this was right up my alley. *I was looking for teenage happiness*, and this play would help me find exactly what I desired. I honestly knew that landing a lead role was improbable, actually, at my size, *impossible.* Lead roles just didn't go to morbidly obese people, at least not in a play all about finding happiness.

When there wasn't enough parts to go around, Mrs. Mason decided to write a few additional scenes and characters into the play. One of those characters was a reporter for *"Sewing Made Easy Magazine,"* who was very interested in the fashion of the bride to be in our happy little production. That reporter had the funniest line in the entire play. The reporter was me and the funniest line in the entire play was completely dependent on my size. And I was completely fine with that dynamic.

The set up was simple. The Happiness Machine paired the perfect couple and the female lead was overjoyed, but the male lead, played by a kid named Kit (see what I mean by the cool name thing?), wanted no part of this mechanically decided romance. When Kit Demus's character rejected Courtney Greer's character—it was Sean Anderson's cue to be instantly famous for the rest of junior high. *"I'll marry her!"* I delivered that line with a big, fat, clumsy enthusiasm that generated a punch like no other. The line, followed by Courtney's sobbing rejection of me, worked for one reason only. I was the fat kid. It worked in front of the entire school and it worked again in front of the parents.

My status in the halls of Stillwater Junior High School was elevated. I was liked, I made people laugh, it didn't get me a girlfriend, *I was still fat,* but people seemed to enjoy me. And *I enjoyed them enjoying me,* even if it meant enthusiastically playing the part of the lovable fat guy. I had become the cool fat kid, and since maintaining that status didn't require me to lose weight, I coasted right along, without a care or thought about my constantly increasing size.

The longer I tried to ignore the obvious growing problem that was my weight, the heavier the topic became when I would finally snap back to reality. I didn't coast careless for very long, before I hatched another wonderful plan to lose the weight once and for all. This time would be the time, I decided. I had spent my entire first year as a teenager wishing I wasn't fat, so now, at fourteen, it was time to do something special. I decided on a set calorie limit and exercise. *Sounds familiar?* On the surface, absolutely, but it was very different than my success today, but identical to numerous failed attempts in my past. It was simply a means to lose weight. Eat less, exercise more, and pretend that everything was fine and dandy along the way.

Admitting I was a food addict and really dealing with my issues was far beyond my fourteen–year-old brain. I just wanted to lose the weight and get a girlfriend, that's it. I wanted to be considered "cute" by the girls in school. I wasn't really trying to change my relationship of dependency and abuse of food, but I was just changing my behavior for the moment. Just long enough to lose weight, but struggling the entire time. I was always one bad day away from throwing in the towel. And that bad day came November 30, 1985 at Yer Mother's restaurant on the world famous Strip in Stillwater.

My family, well, we were bargain hunters. Had to be, because money was always scarce. We could always find the best deals at restaurants. Mainly fast food places, especially if McDonald's was accepting all competitors coupons in exchange for buy-one-get-one free sandwiches. Often times, we would feed all of us: Mom, my little brother Shane, Aunt Kelli, Grandma and Grandpa, and me—for five bucks. *"You can't cook at home that cheap,"* was our mantra.

We were absolute pros at eating out on the cheap long before "value menus" swept the fast-food industry. What does this have to do with Yer Mother's restaurant and November 30, 1985? Yer Mother's wasn't a fast-food place, it was a college hang-out-home-cooking kind of place where homesick college kids could find inexpensive taste of home. *How inexpensive?* On the date in question, it was the infamous ninety-nine-cent chicken fried steak dinner. *"You can't cook at home that cheap!"* You couple that price with my love of chicken fried steak covered in cream gravy, and well, another weight loss attempt was shattered.

I remember the specific date because it was the night of the bedlam game Ice Bowl between OU and OSU. I had over thirty days of continuous weight loss success behind me. Somehow, I held it together that long, and somehow I let it all go that night. The attraction of the dinner was powerful in itself, indeed one of my favorites, and the fact that it was almost free made it impossible to resist. I enjoyed every single gravy-covered bite.

The truth was, it didn't really have to be the end. But in my mind, there was no going back. The next day came and it was like I had never started losing weight. I was completely engulfed in my old behaviors again. *What did they put in that gravy to make me think this way?* What I didn't realize at fourteen was this: It wasn't anything *they* put in the gravy, it was what *I* was putting in my head. This weight loss attempt, like all of the others before it and several after, was as fragile as the thinnest glass. It didn't have to end this way, but to me, it already did. As soon as that gravy hit my tongue, it destroyed the mindset that had carried me this far. I had ruined it. Not really, but you couldn't convince me of the truth back then. I was broken, I was done, and I was stuffed, again.

Maybe being the funny fat guy wasn't such a bad gig after-all. Perhaps, I just needed to relax a little and just not worry about my weight gain and the consequences it created. *Was I ever going to have a girlfriend? Who needs one?* I mean, really, I had a bunch going my way. I had a wonderful family that loved me, my grades in junior high were really decent, except for algebra, and I was generally liked by almost everyone in school. If I ever became stressed or sad, I could stuff those emotions with more gravy, ice cream, pizza, or buy-one-get-one sandwiches from McDonald's, and not feel the least bit stressed about my increasing size. *Why get stressed about it?* I eat when I'm stressed, so I was better off just not worrying about my weight. *There,* that's one less thing to be stressed over.

Teenage romance? Whatever. If it was going to happen, it was going to happen with me just the way I was, because change was something I refused to control at that age. I simply let the changes shape me, adjusting and accepting as needed, good or bad, and trying not to complain along the way. I was choosing this easier way to exist at the line of least resistance. Maybe I could accidentally land a girlfriend back there, I thought. But if I didn't, oh well, their loss. I was going to be somebody someday, and then they'd all be sorry. Never mind that the line of least resistance is probably the last place you want to hang out if you really plan on being somebody, *anybody,* but the me that was being shaped by my casual acceptance of morbid obesity and all of the seriously unfunny limitations included.

I was never comfortable at the line of least resistance. I couldn't accept what it meant, and that was giving up. I didn't really want to give up, unless something became too hard, or stressful, or emotionally overwhelming, then I could retreat back to my comfort zone until that zone became uncomfortable again. It was a cycle of caring *followed by not caring* followed by action and *then inaction.* It was a pattern that was slowly putting me into a very real teenage depression. I knew what I wanted, but I wasn't ready to do what it took to achieve. Maybe I just needed some discipline in my life. Maybe it was time to reignite the spark Mr. McClain was trying to kindle in me, maybe it was time to try out for football.

Chapter Four

Suiting Up

Two-a-days were starting soon, just before my sophomore year, and after a few friends encouraged me to try, I decided to set aside my insecurities and just do the best I could, without stressing over the potential outcome. It might be a wonderful thing, it might work me into shape like I've never known. *Girls like football players, right?* Hey, this could be the answer to everything!

Coach Defee didn't look at me like Mr. McClain did. He could read me like a book, he knew the story: The fat kid with hardly any muscle tone decides he wants to change his life and body, and football is the vehicle that will take him there . . . *if he's willing to work hard.* But this fat kid oozes excuses and whiny behavior. The kid wants *it*, whatever *it* is, but he isn't willing to accept the commitment needed to get there, and Coach Defee doesn't waste time on kids who aren't willing to work.

A slight shift in my attitude, in the way I carried myself into that first day of two-a-days, just a little glimpse of *"I'm not giving up,"* and I think Coach Defee would have been one of my best friends. And I could have been a massive lineman, perhaps worthy of division one looks someday. Instead, my high school football career started and ended the same day, in a very familiar way.

The sun beat down hard on that early August day. It was early in the morning, but already the temperature was flirting with ninety degrees. It was going to break one hundred degrees, and this was the day I picked to not give up. I had zero experience in two-a-days of any kind, unless we're talking about naps. And I had a serious history of walking away from anything difficult. When the coaches decided to run us around the track, I was of course, the slowest out of everyone. Instead of giving me a break, because obviously, I was having the hardest time out there, I was instructed to run another lap. This was hard.

How bad did I want to change? Not enough, because I made a horrible decision at that moment. I decided that when the track curved, I was going to stay straight. And I did. I escaped to the shopping center across the street, ducking into a boot store and pretending to be a shopper. I guess I thought the coaches would come running after me, so I was literally on the run! But the coaches knew, I wasn't ready in any way, to give them, *to give myself*, the kind of commitment needed to survive two-a-days, be on the team, and dramatically change the course of my life. *It was just too hard.*

My grandparents lived less than a quarter mile away, on the other side of the shopping center, and I knew that I was just a few minutes from the peace and comfort of Grandma's sofa, the remote control, and something to eat.

On the way to Grandma and Grandpa's, I really thought I was smart for ducking into the boot store. *They'll never find me in here,* I thought. Never mind that they weren't looking for me to begin with, but I imagine they eventually heard about my little boot shopping excursion in the middle of practice.

You see, they might not have found me, but Mr. Wright did. Mr. Wright was the owner of the boot store and father of two sons, Todd and Tate, both star kickers for Stillwater High. Todd later kicked for Arkansas and Tate for Kansas State. *"Practice over already?"* He asked, and I sheepishly replied, *"No, but it is for me."* Then I quietly and quickly exited his store. It wasn't just practice that was over for me; it was the day that a dream without action *died.*

I let it go that day, the thought that I could change into some kind of in-shape athletic guy, who had zero trouble getting the girls and oozed popularity. *That wasn't going to be me.* I just walked away, disappointed in myself, crushed really, and teetering on the edge of some serious teenage depression.

I don't really remember much about my first sophomore year, except of course, the football experience that preceded. I remember not caring, I remember gaining weight in a very steady fashion, and I remember flunking out of most all my classes. I was a wreck.

When the embarrassment and shame from my bad grades overcame me, I bought blank stolen report cards from a friend and gave myself mostly A's. I remember getting caught when Miss Cook called my mom to talk about my failing English grade and Mom informed her that I had brought home an A, not an F, and there must be some kind of mistake! Oh, there was a huge mistake, alright.

When I discovered that I was caught, I ran once again, across the street, this time checking myself into a cheap motel. I don't remember why I had so much money on me, but I did. Enough to check into the room at the Circle D Motel, lay on the bed, watch Fraggle Rock on HBO, and order a pizza from Domino's.

A large pizza and a nap would make everything better. I was on the run once more, but like a really bad criminal, I made a critical error. I ordered the pizza under my real name. The owner of the Domino's franchise was the father of a friend of mine. He recognized *"Sean Anderson"* on the ticket and immediately called the school.

There I was, relaxing on a motel bed, watching HBO and appreciating the genius puppeteer of Fraggle Rock, trying to forget my troubles, and waiting on a large pizza that would help me escape further into the incredible taste of a melted cheese and mushroom world where troubles no longer existed, only amazing flavor and satisfaction.

I was watching the clock, *are they not supposed to deliver in thirty minutes or less? I just might get this one for free!* When the knock finally came, I heard *"Pizza delivery,"* from a female voice. I quickly opened the door to find Dr. Meritt, the principal of Stillwater High School, and she didn't have a pizza—it was time to face the music I didn't want to hear. *I was busted.*

That school year was a deep dark place I created. Although I probably wouldn't have admitted it at the time, I was severely depressed. I didn't care about anything or anyone. My emotional dependency on food was at an all time high as I wallowed in self-pity, absorbed with being the victim of so many things.

It's amazing what growing older and maturing does for our perspective. In hindsight, I had it really good. Lots of love, plenty to eat, a comfortable place to sleep, great family and friends . . . *I had it all.* But all I could focus on at that age was the negative and the "if only."

If only I would have had a father in my life. If only we wouldn't have been poor. If only my right arm wasn't defective. If only I was naturally thin with a wonderful metabolism, if only I had a pair of leather Kaepa tennis shoes—you know, the ones with dual shoe strings.

If only, if only, if only. The biggest of these was always, *if only* I wasn't fat. Being a normal size, in my mind, was the answer to *everything,* of course, it wasn't then and it isn't now. But in the middle of that state of mind, it was always something or someone that could fix everything, not me, because *I was the victim here, poor me.* I hated being different, being the fat kid, being considered disgusting by the girls. And since changing all of that was just too hard to even imagine accomplishing without someone or something doing it for me, I ran the other way to a place where it didn't matter anymore, and I was able to exist there because of my victim mentality. It wasn't my fault, so why not just accept it and survive, right? If I had discovered that I could choose change, take charge, accept responsibility, and be whatever I wanted, then I wouldn't have been able to live with myself in that self-imposed misery.

Chapter Five

A Short Careless Summer

S urvival by simply existing without regard to the consequences of my bad choices led to many nights of cooking and binging and gaining. This was the road to 505. Giant pots full of mashed potatoes and a big pan of homemade sausage gravy at midnight. Or a few big bowls of ice cream, or sugary sweet cereal, or *"Hey, let's order a pizza!"* Losing weight was the furthest thing from my mind, yet the constant struggle of obesity was always fresh, reminding me of my limitations, keeping me in check, if you will. Whatever good was coming my way had to just happen on its own because I wasn't doing anything but self-destructing.

I needed a fresh start, a clean slate, another chance to make it all right. I needed to care enough to make the most of a re-do, and that's exactly the opportunity the school presented. I had failed so many required classes that I was basically being held back a year. I would get to have a second sophomore year! *Oh boy, lucky me!* Yeah, let's just forget this first sophomore year existed. I was a summer away from a clean slate, a new beginning, a fresh start. I was going to be just fine, *absolutely.* Now, *how about that pizza? We need to celebrate new beginnings!*

A forgettable summer ended quickly and my new opportunity was fresh and exciting. I was fifteen years old, almost 300 pounds, and by all outward appearances—the smiling, big, happy, fat guy. I wasn't even thinking about girls anymore. I had long since given up on the idea of a girlfriend. But everything was about to change.

Section Two

Escape Attempts

"Living my life in denial, I try everything except truth."

Chapter Six

Of Lips and Chickens

My cousin Steve and I enjoyed lunch at Grandy's across the street from the school one day, that first week, when on the way back, a couple of girls yelled for our attention. Steve knew them, he had spent the previous school year at the junior high dodging their flirtations. His attitude of, *oh, brother, not these two,* was completely different than mine. *What do they want?* I wondered. The red headed girl was giggling with the brownish-blond haired one, and then she hollered a question to Steve from sixty yards away. *"Who is that guy with you? What's his name?"* Steve shouted back, *"It's my cousin, Sean."* That's all I needed that day to leave me on cloud nine.

Why were they asking about me? I didn't assume anything. *Are they blind? Why would anyone be interested in me?* I'm grotesquely obese, a freak, *look away, I'm hideous!* Even if all that wasn't true, it's what I felt inside, *it's what I believed.*

When the beautiful brownish blond-haired girl started stepping on my heals in the hall, I was kind of upset. *Why is she picking on me?* I hate it when my heels are stepped on, giving me a "flat tire." She thought it was funny. I thought it was annoying. But when I finally turned around and looked into her smiling eyes, I knew, as hard as it was for me to accept, that she liked me, *uh, that way.*

Again, is she blind? She wasn't blind, but she didn't see what I saw in the mirror. She looked past my physical imperfections and was

43

acting genuinely interested in me. I had to further investigate, for this could be huge. *I want to kiss her!*

Calm down, Sean, be cool, don't act too eager. My self talk must have worked well because she'll tell you to this day that I stood her up for a dance that first week of school. I wasn't acting eager at all. But these two best friends weren't giving up on me very easily.

Irene Brake was Ginger and Rachel Bryant was Cinnamon. They were the original spice girls, long before The Spice Girls came along. So prominent was this spice name thing among them and their friends, I actually thought their names were really Ginger and Cinnamon. And since I was trying to keep four names straight instead of two, I became confused, thinking Irene was Rachel for a little while. This confusion lasted long enough for me to carve *"I love Rachel"* on the wooden desk in my bedroom. I quickly found out who was who. I also quickly forgot about that little affectionate carving. Irene discovered it six months later and I had some serious explaining to do.

Irene gave me her phone number and I looked terrified at her. We didn't have a phone at home. I didn't have a number to give. *Now what? Think fast!* I ended up giving her my Uncle Keith's phone number. Never mind that I was rarely at Keith's apartment, it was a number. I hurried home and immediately told my mom of the situation. *"We have to get a phone, Mom, I have to have a phone number to give this girl!"* We couldn't afford a phone, that's why we didn't have one. A phone was a luxury that we had before, but it became too expensive, and now, if we needed to use a phone, we walked to the pay phone at the apartment laundromat. I couldn't give her a pay phone number, *what would she think of me?* I told Keith she might call and to please just say I wasn't there, and he did several times. *This girl wanted me!* Imagine that. We needed a phone *yesterday.*

I still don't know to this day how Mom did it, but she did it. Within a couple of days, we had a phone number and a phone. She seemed to understand the urgency. I was finally interested in a girl, who was equally interested in me, and Mom was going to help me in any way she could. It wasn't long before I was spending time on the phone with Irene, finally asking her out on our first official date. Friday, September 7th, 1987. Yes, I remember the date! It was a night I'll never forget, even though I couldn't tell you the name of the movie playing, I can tell you that I was feeling an excited nervousness I never knew existed.

It was a double date of sorts. I picked up my cousin Steve in a borrowed Toyota Corolla, and we proceeded to pick up Irene and Rachel, or Ginger and Cinnamon, as they preferred to be called. I wasn't even old enough to drive, I didn't even have a license. I borrowed the car from a college student I worked with at Kentucky Fried Chicken, a job I had just started, and one that I technically wasn't old enough to have, but as you can see, I was an impatient excitable kid who was hell bent on breaking most every rule. If a girl was going to express interest in me, by golly—*nothing was standing in my way of impressing her,* regardless of my age or the law.

We enjoyed burgers and fries at JB's Catfish, a location that today is home to Charlie's Chicken in Stillwater, and we sit in a dark theater and tried to kiss each other, never quite making the connection, we were both too nervous. The movie? I have no idea. It might as well have been called "Ginger Lips," because that's where all my attention was centered.

When the movie ended and we dropped off Steve and then Rachel home, it was just the two of us, *finally.* Irene jumped out of the car when we pulled up to her house. We were running a little late—and she had to go quickly. Her grandparents were not going to be impressed with me and our tardiness. Just when I thought I would have to wait for that kiss I was hoping for all night, she reached back into the car and kissed me, somewhere between my lips and nose. It was perfect and I was mesmerized. She kissed me, *me! Sean Anderson just got kissed by a real live girl!*

.

She didn't care that I was fat and ugly, she didn't see me that way. I was cute and lovable, I was funny, I was wonderful in her eyes. And in my eyes, my passion burned hot for her, stinging in the most wonderful way, turning red with a young love on fire. *Can you believe she kissed me?* It was the beginning of a new world for both of us. A world where growing up was put on fast-forward because we wouldn't have it any other way. And now that I had a girlfriend who loved me despite my size, I was free to get bigger and funnier. But weighing in at over 300 pounds at sixteen wasn't funny to me, and it was downright scary to my mom.

Mom accompanied me to the doctor shortly after my sixteenth birthday. I don't remember the specifics of that doctors visit, except my weight. I had finally topped the scale at just over 300 pounds. I wasn't really that moved over the number. Mom, on the other hand, was horrified at my ballooning out-of-control weight. It was the first of many moments when Mom would plead with me to do something in an effort to lose weight. She was scared for me, *but I wasn't.* I was smitten with Irene and that's all that mattered to me at that time.

"Son, please promise me you'll get busy and try to lose some weight, your weight scares me." That same line was delivered with a sincere concern and horrified worry in 1987, 1997, and 2007, and many other times in between and along the way. My weight was always heavy on Mom's mind and she would often lose sleep obsessing over my increasing number on the scale. As my weight grew, so did her worry. Eventually, she would call me in tears in the middle of the night, practically begging me to "get busy" and lose weight. I would help her sleep by promising to try, but mainly I was just trying to calm her fears long enough to let her rest.

Losing weight was something very hard to do, I was convinced. It was much easier to say that everything would be OK, and *"Someday, Mom, someday I will lose this weight . . . just relax and rest, I feel great, really, it's OK."* Yeah, lying to my mother and myself was much easier than actually trying to do something about my increasing size.

If anyone accused me of being head over heels with Irene simply because she was the first girl who gave me the time of day, I would argue with them. Irene wasn't like the other girls. The other girls looked at me like I was a freak, or at least that's how they made me feel, or maybe it was all in my head and I was the one who looked at me like a freak. All I know is this: My weight, *my looks* didn't matter to Irene. I was cute, *handsome really,* in her eyes. And it was her ability to look past everything that I had concluded the separator between me and teenage happiness, that made me fall in love with the most beautiful girl, inside and out, at Stillwater High School.

Our influence on each other was profound. She grew up in a very sheltered environment, raised and adopted by her grandparents, who had been married young and survived the Great Depression. They were frugal, it was their way of life, an element of survival that guaranteed they would never be without, even if it appeared that they barely had enough. Bertha Brake knew how to stretch a grocery dollar like nobody's business, and they rarely ate out. I was a frequent diner at fast food restaurants far and near. I'm not sure which was bigger, my fascination with having a girlfriend and dating, or Irene's fascination with all of the wonderful restaurants our dating included. We were both experiencing a whole new world, loving it, and loving each other.

It wasn't long before Irene and I were inseparable. If we were in different classes or I was working at Kentucky Fried Chicken, we were still consumed in thoughts of each other. I flunked out of typing class because instead of my regular assignments, I spent class time typing love letters. What did I type? Here's a pretty good example:

Dear Irene,

I love you. I miss you horribly. It's been two hours since I've had a chance to see you, and that's too long. I'm in typing class, just thinking about you and your soft lips. Here comes the teacher . . . Oh, crap, I think she's on to me. Will you still love me if I fail this class? I probably will fail, considering it's taken me twelve minutes to type this. I don't get the "home row" thing, ya know? I can't imagine not looking at the keys and just blindly trusting I'm hitting the right ones. OK, I better wrap this up. I love you! See you at lunch. Pizza and fries? Or do you want a sack of thirty-nine-cent bean burritos from Taco Mayo? I want what you want. Love you!

Yep, we were blindly obsessed with each other, and to me, it was the greatest thing ever.

My behaviors with food didn't improve, they just changed. Instead of eating in a state of depression, I was eating in a state of young love euphoria. When Irene was hired at Kentucky Fried Chicken, we became even more inseparable and gained a bunch of weight together, thanks in part to a manager who was willing to bend the rules a little.

Normally, the leftover food at closing was to be thrown away. But Akbar, the assistant manager, felt the same way we did. *Why let all that good food go to waste?* What's the difference between throwing it all away and carting it off and devouring everything? Akbar would whisper, *"You take whatever you want home, just be quiet about it."* So, at the end of every shift, we loaded up on fried chicken, biscuits, mashed potatoes, gravy, and corn on the cob, repeating the same routine every night after work. The luxury of KFC, normally something we only enjoyed at family reunions and special occasions, became a "three to four night a week" ritual. We would pack it all in and head to a picnic area, eat until we were absolutely stuffed sick, then exchange greasy kisses all night long.

Everything was right with the world at that point. It was because we made our entire world all about each other. We forgot that we were still kids, opting instead for a fast track to adulthood and adult responsibilities. Losing weight was the furthest thing from my mind during this pivotal time. We were focused on our relationship. I provided an escape for Irene and she provided one for me. A girlfriend, a real girlfriend, *finally!* And I didn't have to lose the weight, or become a football star, or anything other than just being me.

As our focus on each other grew, everything else suffered. We both neglected our school work, our families, and even our friends. Ours was a twenty-four-seven relationship. If we weren't together, we were on the phone. If we were together, nothing else mattered. Young love, boldly proceeding without a firm grip on reality, just a firm grip on each other. We worked together, we ate together, we were inseparable. My little brother Shane was quickly reaching an age when he could have used my big brotherness, but I wasn't available. Irene's little sister, JoEllen, probably could have used Irene's big sisterness, but again—we only made time for each other. We did everything together. And out of everything we did, the thing we did most, was dream of a better life . . . and having kids. Crazy, huh? Kids dreaming of having kids. Isn't having kids at such a young age supposed to be accidental? It wasn't with us. We planned it all. We dreamed it before it happened. And while most of our dreams were without any clue of how to accomplish them, the having a baby dream, was easy. We just had to do what teenagers with raging hormones do, except we did it without regard to consequences.

Chapter Seven

Hiding Behind a Microphone

If I was going to fast forward into adulthood, I needed a career. I would often listen to the radio and dream of being a disc jockey. In the summer of my sixteenth year, I decided to act on the dream. I composed a letter to Dave Collins, the program director of KVRO radio in Stillwater. I wish I had that letter today, because it was good!

I told Dave how I wanted to be in broadcasting as a career and how I planned on going to school for it someday. I told of how I wanted to get a head start and learn everything I could, and that I would even work for free if he couldn't pay me. It wasn't a week after I dropped off that letter, when the phone was ringing with that smooth voice on the other end, asking if I could come in for an interview. *Wow—this is my big chance,* I thought. I was young, disillusioned, and eager to do or say whatever was necessary to get hired.

Dave made the interview so easy. I was a big kid with a big smile and he knew, if given the chance, I would be the most loyal employee he could ever want. He hired me on the spot and even agreed to pay me! *Wow—I'm going to get paid to be a disc jockey? At sixteen? How cool is this?* And the station was a Top Forty format, so all of my friends listened. I was about to become a local celebrity with a career track starting at sixteen!

How much was I going to make? I said I would do it for free, but when he said that he couldn't do that, and that he would pay me, my mind came up with all kinds of wonderful figures. My illusions were shattered when he revealed that minimum wage, three thirty-five an hour would be the pay rate.

Oh, well, the experience was more valuable than any amount of money! I was assigned to operate the Rick Dees Weekly Top Forty program on the weekends. This sounded huge to me. My illusions were once again shattered when I found out that this simply meant playing the program off of vinyl 33 1/3 RPM records and playing the local commercials when directed. *But when do I get a chance to talk on the air?* Dave told me to wait until I was ready. I guess he didn't understand my impatient personality.

I'm pretty sure that Dave had planned to tell me when I was ready to crack the microphone, but I wasn't waiting. A couple of months into the job, at two in the morning on a Sunday, I made my debut. I cherry picked all of my favorite songs while putting on a show and recording the entire thing. I was horrible. But I didn't know. I thought I was amazing. I quickly rushed home and made a bunch of duplicate cassettes to send out to every relative and acquaintance I knew. I was officially somebody. And it was perfect. You couldn't see me on the radio, I could look like anything a listener imagined. Suddenly, I realized that this career choice was exactly what I needed to further remove me from caring about my ever expanding size. As long as I could talk, I could put on a show, entertain, and never feel the insecurities of my appearance. Unless of course the station sent me out to do a broadcast somewhere, then I would have to face people. But that was still a ways away in my young career.

I really thought I had successfully hijacked the station on that early Sunday morning without anyone being the wiser. I knew I didn't have permission, but I didn't care. In my mind, I was so good that, even if Dave heard me, he would quickly realize that I was a natural, and needed to be on the air as much as possible. Unfortunately, Dave didn't see it that way. And he was listening, and he didn't react even remotely close to what I had hoped. He called me at home and ordered me to the station for a talk.

Dave had planned on firing me. I had disregarded his direction and took over the radio station to do an unauthorized broadcast. But something stopped him from getting rid of me. Maybe he could see that this and a girlfriend was all I had, all I wanted. It was my world.

He told me, *"Don't you ever crack the mic again without my permission, if you do, you're out!"* Wow—that was a close call. I had one other brush with a near firing when he pulled up on Christmas day, and instead of being in the studio baby-sitting thirty-minute reel to reel blocks of Christmas music, I was outside in the street passing a football back and forth with my cousin Steve. Dave wasn't amused or understanding in the least. Good thing he didn't fire me because I had left my head cook position at Kentucky Fried Chicken to pursue radio exclusively.

It was a very content time for me. I had a girlfriend, the coolest job for a teenager, ever, and I hadn't a care about much else. I wasn't really concerned with my weight. I was concerned with very little. I didn't care about school, my weight, my family, friends, anyone or anything. It was Irene and radio, and a comfortable ignorance from reality. I didn't think about my weight again until a radio sales rep approached me about Nutri-System.

The deal was simple. I would get the Nutri-System plan for free, in exchange for talking about how wonderful it was on the radio. My attitude was one of, *OK, let's see if this works.* It needed to do it for me, completely, because I wasn't anywhere ready to do anything. With this new plan, I started to think about what it might be like to lose the weight. I hadn't thought of losing weight in a while—and the number on the scale showed. I was above 400 pounds. I swear, the time it took to go from three hundred to four, was seriously, maybe six to nine months. I was out of control in so many ways.

My counselor at Nutri-System told me all about the program, gave me bags of food and the plan, and sent me on my way. All I had to do was eat exactly what was in my plan and the weight would melt away.

The food was horrible, especially the dehydrated hamburger and the mini-pizza. But you couldn't tell on the air. *It was the most wonderful thing! The food tasted great and I was losing weight so easily!* But the truth was simple: I hated every day. I hated the food and I hated the accountability of the weigh-ins and the on-air reports of my success or failure. Failing really wasn't an option because I had to succeed— Nutri-System was a client, and if I screwed this up, it could mean my job. Lucky for me, the client ended up canceling their advertising contract and I was off the hook and back to eating whatever I wanted and as much as I wanted. I was so glad that was over. *And people actually pay big money for that stuff?* I wasn't ready to do anything for myself. And the little bit of weight I did lose, came roaring back, plus some, as soon as I returned to my food addict behaviors that brought me to over 400 pounds at seventeen.

Chapter Eight

Living in Fast Forward

I really didn't have time to focus on losing weight anyway. I was getting ready to ask Irene to marry me. Well, we were together all the time anyway, we might as well be husband and wife, right? This was the logic my grandmother shared, and I used it almost word for word in my proposal. It was quite possibly the most unromantic proposal in the history of proposals: *"Uh, Irene, uh, my grandma thinks we spend so much time together that we should just get married. You want to get married?"* I didn't get on one knee or anything. I just delivered it in the same casual tone as, *"Hey, you wanna go grab a pizza?"* Despite the horrible proposal that would never be forgotten, and often thrown up in arguments or casual conversations with friends (I don't blame her), she said yes! We were set. We were getting married and starting an adult life together. The date was set: April 16th, 1989.

While all of the other kids our age were busy with high school, planning for college, and living normal teenage lives, we were caught up in some kind of disillusioned dream land, where nobody could change our mind with reason. Momma tried, but I wasn't listening. Irene's grandparents tried to talk some sense into us, too, but again— we knew what was best for us.

We seemed to know that if we were ever going to learn anything, it was going to be the hard way because we wouldn't allow any other way. That same method of learning the hard way would be repeated over and over, in everything we did, including weight-loss attempts.

Who has time to think about weight loss? We were trying to plan a wedding, a family, manage a broadcasting career, and trying to figure out the quickest and least embarrassing way to flunk out of all our classes.

It must have been tough for my mom and other family members to watch. We were like a runaway train, you couldn't stop us. We were bent on doing things our way. And somehow, we convinced everyone to just agree and go along with us. Looking back now, I can't believe some of the crazy things we did and experienced so young. It was a heck of a way to learn about life, but for us, *it was the only way.*

The fast forward button was pressed and stuck, headed straight for adulthood. I was comfortably over 400 pounds when we married. Comfortable, as in, well, over 400 pounds. I wasn't physically comfortable, ever.

The outfit I wore for the wedding was horrendous. Somewhere, there's pictures. It's really bad. Anyway, we didn't waste any time at all when it came to starting a family because Amber was conceived on our honeymoon night. We know because that was the only time we were not *"careful."* I'm sure that some who attended our wedding probably thought we were expecting, and that's why we were getting married so young. When Irene started showing signs of the pregnancy, they were convinced, I'm sure. But no, not at all. We were in love and we were planning our future. *Relax, we knew what we're doing! Yeah, right!*

We were a little too relaxed. When Irene's water broke on the morning of January 4th, 1990, we casually celebrated. Irene took time to fix her hair and we drove over to her grandma and grandpa's house to tell them, *this was the day!* After cruising around town a while, we finally made our way to the hospital where Amber would come along at 12:19 PM.

I snapped a bunch of pictures in the delivery room. I have no idea what happened to those photos, maybe they were destroyed. These pictures were graphic, nothing anyone in their right mind would want to show around. But I clearly wasn't in mine, so I did, showed them around, to everyone. Irene could have killed me and she would have been justified. I was just so happy to be a new dad. It was an intoxicating feeling. I was drunk with stupidity, completely unprepared and careless.

When Irene expressed a desire for some non-hospital food, I quickly made my way to McDonald's where a friend of mine was the manager. It was closing time and they had a bunch of sandwiches left over. Upon hearing the good news, my friend loaded me up with sacks full of everything. I carried enough McDonald's back to Irene's room to feed a dozen people. We gorged on our favorites and marveled at the newborn that we had brought into our insane little world.

The same time we were dealing with the self-imposed pressures of married life and starting a family, I went straight into another storm of emotions. I decided that it was time to find my dad.

I believe we all have an emotional limit, and I was seriously about to find mine. I wasn't happy with myself in so many ways, and this was another attempt to "heal" me and find some happiness. I was many years from realizing the truth that happiness must come from within, and so I continued living beyond my years with a blissful ignorance in my search.

A bunch of the happenings and pivotal events consumed the next year or so in my life, ones I would rather forget. I had an emotional and mental breakdown that included loading up my mom's Chevy Chevette with Irene, Amber, and a childhood of questions and resentment, and trying to drive to meet my dad for the first time, only to turn around within one hundred miles of his house, and heading back home.

On the way back home, in the middle of my emotional and mental breakdown, we stopped to help a family who were mechanically broke down, and ended up being robbed and held against our will. This was the very last thing we needed at that moment. If it hadn't been for Irene's strength and courage, who knows what would have happened. We had guardian angels for sure, no doubt.

It was Irene, Amber, and me in a very bad situation that was getting worse by the hour. It's a very long story that ended when Irene realized that I hadn't the emotional energy left to safely get us out of the situation. The leader of this "gang" had his eye on Irene, and plans to dump me in the Mississippi River were spoken where she could hear. It was scary to Irene, but I wasn't understanding the threat like she was, with her in her right mind, and me in the middle of a nervous breakdown.

And Amber was too young to realize what was happening, thank goodness. Irene had to rise up and rescue our young family and that's exactly what she did. She took charge and we escaped that horrible dwelling in Oceola, Arkansas without any of us being killed, although Irene was assaulted at one point. I was so mentally exhausted. We needed serious help. I needed serious professional help, the comfort of home, and rest from the chaos created.

When we arrived safely back at Mom's house, we felt the comfort and calm that was settled in that apartment. Mom prepared us a hot meal, Hamburger Helper Cheeseburger Macaroni if I remember right, and I do, because it was the best tasting Hamburger Helper I'd ever eaten. I remember every bite to this day. I'm not saying that I was feeding my emotions, not at all. In this case, after all we had endured, it was a combination of peace, safety, love, and the best tasting cheeseburger macaroni in the world. We were home, but I was still having serious trouble emotionally.

I often think about how wonderful it could have been to lose the weight at this young age. But with everything else in our lives creating a constant chaotic desperation, there just wasn't time or energy to devote to anything but survival.

Chapter Nine

Waiting for Change

My choices brought me to a dark place where I honestly felt powerless to make the changes needed to lose weight. What were those changes, anyway? I mean, come on—I had found love, married, became a father, landed in an exciting career, and reached out to the father I never knew.

None of these changes provided the motivation or inspiration that I needed to make me "click." I had given up hope of ever changing. Still, somewhere deep inside, I hoped that change could come and save me. It had to be some monumental event that would come along out of the blue, swoop in and fix everything.

If losing weight was ever to become a priority, it would have to jump up and get my attention . . . and it was about to, several times.

At well over 400 pounds, any little twinge of chest pain would send me into a state of panic. It was like a sudden reminder, a jolt of reality, a sudden death looming if I didn't do something soon. I remember one time in particular, when the pain in my chest, and my out of control obesity, made me feel like I was on death's door. We rushed to the emergency room and it wasn't long before I was hooked up to all kinds of monitors.

I hated every second of the process because it meant taking off my shirt so they could apply the EKG leads. Irene was right by my side, tears in her eyes, trying not to think about my over-worked heart succumbing to the pressures of a 450-pound body. This time, like many more to come, I was convinced that my time was up.

Right there in the emergency room bed, I would proclaim my devotion to change. This was it. I would serve up a dying man's prayer to be saved. I was promising God, Irene, and me that things were going to change, if only I could survive this brush with death. I was going to once and for all lose the weight, and *get right by everything.* And in the middle of this last prayer for healing and a second chance, the doctor came in with the news: "Your heart is in great shape. Probably anxiety, and maybe too much caffeine. The EKG looks normal, so you're free to go!" *Wow, really? You mean, I'm not going to die?* Was this an answer to my prayer, or an excuse to keep on not caring? Or both?

As soon as I learned that my heart was still in good shape, I quickly forgot about my promise and plans to get healthy and lose the weight once and for all. It was one less thing to worry about in a life where we created many things to worry about, like how to pay the bills and survive as a too-young family. Let's celebrate, *I'm going to live!*

That insane process would repeat over and over. And when doctors would remind me that eventually my body would have enough, and these tests would start looking bad, it still wouldn't deter me. I was never afraid of death until I thought it was imminent. Irene came to the conclusion years ago, judging from this track record, that someday it would be too late. And oh, *what a sad day that would be*, indeed. But until the next close call, I would just eat my way through everything, eventually developing some serious habits of deceitful eating, or sneak eating. When I started to realize how much my obesity worried my family, that's when I started really hiding the worst of my food addict and compulsive eating behaviors. If I had a quarter for every convenience store deli burrito and corn dog I've consumed in the privacy of my vehicle, *just because,* well—I would be wealthy.

The dependency on food in every situation was always a continuously running behavior for me. Call it habit, or whatever, at a certain point, I couldn't even tell you why I was compelled to eat five bucks worth of Taco Bell on the way to a home cooked meal. It doesn't make sense. I loved the taste of food. That's what I would tell myself. *I loved the taste.* Well, that's simple and not abnormal. Most people love the taste of food. *I just loved it extra special.* But I knew it was wrong, my behaviors with food were completely out of control, and the fact that I would often hide my binging from Irene, tells you that I knew, this was a little more than just a simple love of food.

I became very good at being morbidly obese. I adapted very well to the increasing restrictions I created. If we were dining out, we knew where we could go and where we couldn't. We couldn't go anywhere with small booths or fixed seating of any kind. If their chairs had arms, we were headed somewhere else. Many times, when trying someplace new, we would walk in, scan the dining room, realize that I couldn't fit comfortably, turn around and walk out. There wasn't an explanation offered, just a quick exit. I'm sure the restaurant staff usually knew exactly what was happening. Although, many a hostess tried to seat us in small booths over the years. How embarrassing to explain that "I can't fit *there*, we'll need a table with chairs, and uh, no arms!"

Clothes shopping had long since become a challenge at this point. It was just a given, that if I needed clothes, we would need to load up the car and head toward Oklahoma City or Tulsa, to the nearest Casual Male Big and Tall. It was such a big inconvenience and an expensive necessary alternative. Almost every trip would hear me say, "Someday I'll lose this weight and these trips will be a thing of the past." Probably the first four or five times, Irene believed me when I would utter those same tired words. After awhile, I'm not sure she heard it anymore. Statements like that almost became laughable. It was just something I would say to make myself feel good at the moment, pretending that there was hope for change, but never intending to really do anything concrete to make it happen. Besides, who had time to think about losing weight, when we needed to figure out a good place to eat dinner in the big city! Yeah, I was adapting and accepting my morbid obesity and often times feeling sorry for myself.

I can remember thinking to myself, many times over the years, *why me? Why do I have to be that guy? Why must I be different?* Instead of trying to do something about my weight, I would opt for sitting around thinking about how unfair it was that naturally slim people could eat whatever they wanted, as much as they wanted, and never worry about weight, clothing options, or where they were going to sit in a restaurant. Slim people who have never experienced obesity, those people can eat excessively in public, and nobody gives it a second thought. In fact, if anything is said, it's complimentary. *"That guy can eat, wow! He can really put it away!"* I was jealous of these big eating slender people. *I want a metabolism like that!* I was always quick to feel sorry for myself, but never really that motivated to do something to change.

Our young marriage and family were struggling at best. The medical issues that were becoming more pronounced with my increasing size were starting to take their toll on everyone, and especially Irene. At nearly 500 pounds, my sleep apnea symptoms were raging, but I was undiagnosed at that point. I was just tired all the time. I also had been fighting a long time problem of nighttime bed wetting. When I say I was a mess, I mean literally, in every way. How we stayed together so long, I don't know. If I wasn't working, I was snoring loudly and urinating uncontrollably almost every night. If I were a dog, I'd have been dropped at the pound years ago.

The bed wetting, although extremely personal and embarrassing to share (and something I've never mentioned in the blog), was something that was corrected with a single prescription of a nasal spray. Irene endured years and years of that problem, and with one simple prescription, it finally stopped, forever. If you know of someone suffering from nighttime incontinence, ask a doctor about the nasal spray medication options. It worked for me.

I can't believe I just revealed my past bed-wetting problem. It was something that plagued me as a kid and just never went away, until that one single prescription. I share it, in hopes that someone suffering silently, like I did, will ask for a prescription that could end that horrible disorder in their lives. I also share it, in an effort to properly explain just how miserable everything had become.

I always thought of losing weight as the great corrector of everything bad in my life, but still, I wasn't breaking free anytime soon. I guess I was waiting for the doctor to have some kind of magical prescription, like the nasal spray, that would instantly and permanently rid me of my morbid obesity. Maybe someday that miracle would become reality, I mean, really—surely somewhere, in a lab, scientists are busy trying to create an obesity vaccine. It's funny and sad, some of the crazy day dreams that I entertained at my heaviest.

The one thing that did make my life easier was the fact that I had a talent for radio. I have no idea what I would have done without radio. It made me feel good, it was my career, it's what I did. And it was respected, admired, it was a prestigious job despite the horrible small-market pay. At one point, in 1993, I was bringing home six hundred dollars a month and a rent-free apartment. As long as we were eating and I was on the air, everything was fine for a little while, at least.

In the summer of 1993, Courtney came along. This time, we didn't waste any time in getting to the hospital. Irene woke me up in the middle of the night. She was having contractions. After a few false alarms in the days leading up to July 20th, I was convinced Irene could just go back to sleep and the contractions would go away. It was lazy wishful thinking. Irene knew it was time and as soon as I saw the fear on her face, I knew that this was different than the first.

Something was wrong. We sped all the way to the hospital in a frantic rush. Upon our arrival, the emergency room team quickly examined Irene and determined that it wouldn't be long before delivery. The doctor came in and, after a quick exam, announced the baby was breach. An emergency Caesarean was the only safe option. Things started to get really scary at this point. The anesthesiologist was paged to come in for this middle of the night Caesarean, but they never answered the call. The baby wasn't waiting any longer. The doctor ordered me out of the delivery room and informed us that he would need to attempt a regular delivery of this breach baby.

I was in the waiting room all alone, praying as hard and fast as I knew how. I didn't care if it was a boy or girl, I just wanted Irene and our new baby to be safe and alive. Just as my intense prayer reached its peak, and I said amen, the nurse came in and told me all was well. She invited me to the nursery window to see my new daughter. A girl. Cool! We didn't have an ultrasound early, so it was a surprise. I don't think I've ever had a prayer answered so quickly before or since.

Our family was growing and so was the pressure to lose weight. My concern about the weight would come in waves. I would be really concerned for a very short time, then I would forget about it for a very long time, followed by an occasional awakening from chest pain, or something crazy, like a spider bite.

I swear, a was bitten by a brown recluse spider, and that's what crippled my lymphatic system in my right leg. That's what I've always believed. I still have the discoloration around the area of the bite. So now, my obesity was becoming an even harder situation because my leg was swelling horribly from lymphedema, I was years away from that magic nasal spray that ended my bed wetting, and I was always tired because of raging and undiagnosed sleep apnea. Still, with everything, I was lucky. Whenever it was checked, my blood work looked great. No sugar issues, no cholesterol issues, and surprisingly, it would be over ten years later before I started having high blood pressure problems. Somehow, my problems were not enough to make me want to do anything to turn it all around. And as I said, to me, that was the answer to everything. I just needed to lose the weight, and everything would magically become Disney-like perfect. But even with that belief, I wasn't turning anything around.

I did the best job I knew how to do because I just knew that our way out depended on my ability to put together a good air-check audition tape. This was radio. My education didn't make a difference. It was all in my on-air talent. *What could I do? How talented was I? What did I sound like?* Those were the questions program directors wanted to know. Not, *how much does he weigh?* Or, *what does he look like?* It was all about what was coming through those speakers. *Or so I thought.*

We were surviving. I needed a better job with better pay, in a bigger market. Freedom was just one big break away and until then, euphoria was available at every meal, and if needed, between meals, too.

Chapter Ten

Too Big for Big Time

It didn't take long for our dream of a better life to start happening. The phone call I received from a program director at a big Fort Smith station told me what I already knew. *I had talent.* He listened to my tape, called me, and offered me a job site unseen, over the phone. It was for an over-night air-shift, full-time and more money than I had ever made in radio. *We were going to make it!* This was big news for our young family. Finally, things were looking up! My tape was so impressive to this guy, he didn't even need a face-to-face interview.

My air-check audition tape was bound to get some attention. It was a morning of me doing two morning shows on two different stations at the same time. The owner of the two stations had both wired through the same broadcast console. All I had to do was flip a switch and flip my personality a little, to go from a soft adult-contemporary station on the FM dial to a classic country station on the AM dial. It was something like this, with a soft-toned delivery: *"Seven thirty-seven on Star One-Oh-Five Point One, I'm Sean in The Morning. It's forty seven degrees, on our way to seventy-three. Here's Elton John."* Flip the switch, and the relaxed country style delivery: *"Seven thirty-eight at Star Country Ten-Twenty. We're almost to fifty, and we're not a stoppin' till we hit seventy-three this afternoon. We should cook out, that's nice! Here's a little Willie, on Star Country."*

I couldn't believe the blessing of it all and I couldn't wait to tell Irene of our good fortune. Irene was very excited about moving to Fort Smith. We both had that excited-nervous feeling that comes before big change. We didn't have much, so all we needed was a small U-Haul trailer hitched to our big orange Chevrolet Caprice station wagon to carry everything we owned down I-40, toward the promise of a brand new life in Arkansas. Courtney wasn't even two, and Amber was four, and this was the longest road trip they had ever endured. Amber loved every second. This was exciting to this little girl. Courtney wasn't doing as well. She insisted that Irene turn around from the front seat and hold her hand all the way to Fort Smith. It was fine because nothing could cloud our joy.

As we approached Fort Smith, I tuned in this wonderful new radio station and was absolutely thrilled at what I was hearing. This station sounded amazing to me, and I was going to be one of the jocks! Irene could tell that I was on top of the world happy and excited about this new job. It was all smiles, all the way into Fort Smith and the little downtown motel we would call home for a few days until we could find a place to live. The more Fort Smith we discovered, the more excited we became. From where we came, this was a big city! *We were arriving!*

I had an appointment the next morning to meet the program director and go over the training schedule. I don't remember having any insecurity issues at all that morning. I was confident in my abilities, my talent, and the fact that I was nearly 500 pounds just didn't seem to matter at that point. I quietly left Irene and the girls, along with Irene's sister JoEllen, and JoEllen's daughter, Mary, at the motel while I attended to business. I remember the drive to the station and just being in awe of the city, the traffic, and the radio station where I would call home. It was a real happiness that completely engulfed me in every way.

I pulled up to the station with the U-Haul still attached. I walked inside with a seemingly unshakable confidence. It was short-lived euphoria because I was about to feel something strange. I introduced myself to the receptionist as the "new guy," and was greeted with a straight-faced response. She called the program director in to meet me and immediately I was consumed with that strange-awkward feeling of something wasn't quite right. The program director didn't seem happy to see me. At first I couldn't really pin-point the source of my gut feeling, but as he introduced me to the air-staff, I started noticing a style that wasn't me.

Everyone looked the part. Wranglers and boots and the slickness of a new country artist was the style and vibe of several I met that day. I didn't wear Wranglers and boots on my nearly five hundred pound body, that wasn't me. And this station, I was told, was heavy on personal appearances. I was hired to do over-nights, but was told that part of the job was doing appearances during the morning show. This wasn't going to be the type of job where I could hide behind the microphone, letting the listener decide what I looked like. No, they were going to see me out and about, all over town. And the program director continued the tour with a less than thrilled attitude.

I left the station with an uneasy feeling, but at the same time I knew that all I needed to do was be myself, do a great job on the air, and everything was going to be fine. If the program director had any reservations, I would quickly put his mind to rest with my talent and presentation. I was going to sound great on this station, and to me, that's all that mattered. I was optimistic. My internal hope mechanism was working over time. We were going to make it, despite this feeling I carried back to the little downtown Fort Smith motel. I wasn't about to share my gut feelings with Irene. It was going to work out and I didn't want to worry her needlessly. That night, I returned to the station to train with the guy I was replacing.

The next morning, we picked up a paper and started looking for a place to live. It was just a few hours into our search when we discovered a wonderful apartment community that seemed thrilled to offer an apartment to the latest disc jockey at what I was quickly discovering was the most popular station in town. All we had to do was tell them of my new job, and despite the fact that we were a few hundred dollars short of having enough for the move-in expenses, they gave us a key. We didn't have any furniture, but we didn't care. This was our new home. Furniture would come eventually. I was just happy to be able to unload the U-Haul trailer. The girls were loving our new place, and Irene and I were finally seeing it all come together. We had already paid for the motel room, so with a new lease signed on an empty apartment, we decided to stay one more night downtown.

My next training session was scheduled for that night, but the schedule would change when I called the station to check on the scheduled time. The program director wanted me to come in right away. He had something he needed to talk with me about and he didn't seem to be in a joyful mood. I headed to the station with a rumbling inside. I knew something was up and I feared it wasn't good. I was right.

The program director informed me that the overnight guy had decided to stay. The full-time job I was hired to do was no longer available, but he was happy to offer me a part-time hourly weekend shift instead. I was confused. The guy whom I was replacing, the one who trained me the night before, he was excited to be moving on to bigger and better things. *And now he was staying?* It didn't make sense. I wanted to cry right in front of him. And I had several reasons to be upset. We spent too much money on a U-Haul trailer, way more than we could afford on the motel room, and now we had depleted our funds and signed a lease on an apartment we couldn't possibly keep.

And now—with no full-time air shift, no salary, no security, no insurance, nothing—I had to go back and tell Irene the horrible news. But what really made me feel like weeping was the underlying, unspoken truth of the situation. I wasn't the image they needed and wanted. I was a morbidly obese young man, loaded with talent *that didn't matter* because I didn't fit. I could have been the greatest radio personality of all time and the outcome would have been the same. My morbid obesity had finally busted my internal hope mechanism. I was broken and broke, and extremely scared. I had learned a hard lesson: Talent can only carry you so far when you weigh nearly 500 pounds. Unfortunately, I had taken my whole family along for the ride.

This was discrimination, pure and simple. But it was perfectly acceptable. *Why?* Because radio is part of the entertainment industry. And being discriminated against because of your appearance is part of this industry. I really didn't think this type of thing applied to radio; after all, this industry, with its sedentary working environment, is full of obese people. But in this case, at this station, it did apply. Just as an actor wouldn't get a part he didn't "look right" for, I wasn't going to be a full-time personality on this station because I didn't look right. I was demoted to an overnight weekend part-time announcer who would never do personal appearances. Instead, I would be hidden away in a studio, far away from the public, and I knew that the consolation of a part-time job came as pity, since I had moved my family. Keeping me employed in some way was like an act of compassion from this program director, who probably never again hired someone sight-unseen.

So once again I had big news to tell Irene. Only this time, I wasn't excited and the nervous feeling came from knowing I was about to crush the world of the only woman who ever loved and had faith in me. Her look of joy instantly transforming into a sad desperation, left me feeling scared, hopeless, and completely empty. There we were, standing in an empty apartment, a few pictures already on the wall in what was supposed to be our happy new home. Tears were building in her eyes, and that's all it took for my emotions to overflow. The girls played on the floor in the corner, oblivious to the circumstances. *What now?* We had less than forty dollars to our name. We stood there crying, and as I held her in my arms, a thought formed in my mind. Just across town by the mall, I had seen a Pizza Inn with an all-you-can-eat buffet. I wanted to fill this emptiness the only way I knew how. Within twenty minutes, we were seated at a table with chairs, no arms, and for a few moments, all was right with the world, and then Courtney became sick, throwing up all over the restaurant and snapping us back to the sad reality this entire move had become.

Chapter Eleven

Five Hundred Pounds and Homeless

W hen you're broke, I mean really broke, you do what you must to survive. It didn't take long for us to take a personal inventory and make our way to the rough side of town. This kind of desperation was nothing new around here, and sadly, nothing new to us. Pulling up to the pawn shop in search of some quick cash was something we promised each other we wouldn't ever do again, but here we were, and the gold bands on our fingers were the only things left to liquidate.

Irene slid hers off and handed it to me without looking up. This was the lowest, a cheapening of our vows, neither of us wanted, but it seemed like one of the only options. I had time to think about where we were and what we were doing, while I waited in line. The thirty-five bucks paid for the symbols of our marriage was just enough to get Irene and the girls back to Stillwater, and as disappointing as it was, we knew it had to be the plan. We didn't have enough time and money to improve our situation.

It's not like we didn't try anything and everything to stay. We originally decided to make this work. A lease was signed and Fort Smith would be our new home despite the unfortunate turn of events. Irene immediately started looking for a job and I started investigating every other radio station in the area, in hopes of landing on my feet somewhere. Irene quickly secured a job working the graveyard shift at a convenience store close to the apartment. The EZ Mart would help us make rent and if it came right down to it, I would get some kind, any kind of non-radio job to help make ends meet. This wasn't going to be easy, but we had to make the best of the situation.

The truth about the side of town we called home and the EZ Mart job wasn't good. Irene was scared to death, every night. EZ Marts were getting robbed at gun point all over town, and we knew, it was a matter of time before Irene's life would be in danger. It was simply an intolerable situation. In the meantime, I was interviewing at a variety of non-radio related jobs, but still having zero luck in the search. When Irene came home and described the terror she felt with several late night customers, that was it, she wasn't going back to the EZ Mart. We didn't have much time to get on our feet because our money was gone, rent was due, and we were absolutely desperate.

With pale white circles on our ring fingers and just enough gas in the tank of our bright orange station wagon to get us back to Stillwater, we headed out of Fort Smith feeling horribly defeated. But still, I just couldn't give up. Mom gave me enough money to send me back alone. It was one last attempt to salvage what was supposed to be a wonderful new chapter in our young family's life. Without Irene and the girls, I was supposed to focus on turning it all around, but my focus was distracted by my quickly deteriorating circumstances.

Eventually, the eviction notice came, and I was left sleeping in the car. I would go from one church parking lot to another every night. I took sponge baths in convenience store bathrooms, and when I couldn't take it anymore, I sought refuge at the Salvation Army homeless shelter. This was how far we had fallen. And I knew, it was all because of my morbid obesity. Knowing this obvious truth wasn't ever enough to make me want to lose weight. As an emotional eater, these circumstances sent me running to food even faster, further compounding the problem. I was nearing the end of my rope in so many ways. The shelter was a scary place to me. I was scared, hurt, depressed, and quickly becoming even more of an emotional wreck. I wasn't having any luck in my job search and I was down to my last twenty dollars when another decision was made.

I was going home, defeated and tired. My cousin Travis, just a teenager at the time, wired me enough money to get home. This was my rock-bottom. That drive out of Fort Smith was a tough one to make and I couldn't help but to daydream how it might have been different had I been a normal weight and looked good in a pair of Wranglers and boots.

Chapter Twelve

Living on Tulsa Time

My mom and little brother Shane didn't mind that we were all crowding them in their small one-bedroom apartment. We were surrounded by love and understanding, supported by family, and clinging tight to our hopes and dreams despite the temporary setback of Fort Smith.

I quickly sent out new air-check tapes and it wasn't long before I landed an interview with Star 103 in Tulsa. I always wanted to work in that building. Star 103 was right down the hall from the legendary KRMG and the studio was right next door to K95 FM. These were stations I dreamed of working for, and now I had a chance to be there! It was time to impress in this upcoming interview. This was my time. Who needs Fort Smith? I'm headed to Tulsa!

My experiences in Fort Smith left me feeling ultra aware and super self-conscious about my appearance. Lucky for me, from the moment I met the smiling face of Program Director Jeff Couch, I knew that I needn't worry. He treated me with respect, kindness, and like "one of the guys." Jeff could tell that radio was a passion for me, like it was for him. We were brothers in that way. We were in the same club and I was seriously being considered for a full-time position on the hot new radio station in Tulsa and it didn't matter that I was nearly 500 pounds. This was how it was supposed to be.

I ended up getting beat out by another guy for the full-time position, but Jeff wanted me on staff anyway. I was hired. And I knew that this time, my size had nothing to do with the outcome. I had an opportunity in Tulsa. I would have to find something to supplement my income at Star 103, but I was in the building. I had a chance to prove myself alongside the most talented radio people in the entire state. It was a confidence booster that I carried all the way back to Stillwater and Irene and the girls. We were Tulsa-bound.

Maybe because I was full of confidence or maybe because I was already hired by the most respected broadcast company in town, I don't know, but getting that second supplemental job was easy. I was immediately hired by a studio that produced on-hold messages for companies all over the nation, oh, and they also originated live syndicated via-satellite radio talk shows.

Part of my duties was being the producer for *Health Talk with Becky Dixon.* Becky never confronted me directly about my morbid obesity, but she did indirectly, by occasionally choosing topics that zeroed in on the health risk and dangers of being overweight. There I was, nearly 500 pounds, sitting on the other side of the glass from the host, producing a radio show all about good health and happiness. Occasionally, Becky would look my way while making a sharp point, and I swear she was hoping that I was listening. I probably wasn't. Instead, I found the irony of the situation quite humorous. Besides, I was too busy trying to decide what fast-food place to visit on my way home. Tulsa had choices, endless choices! *A food addict's dream, that city, oh my.*

What would it be today? A giant cream cheese everything bagel from New York Bagel or a bean burrito with sour cream from Taco Bell, or how about a Quarter Pounder with cheese and fries? *This wasn't dinner.* This was a continuously increasing habit I was developing and one that I tried in so many ways to hide from Irene and the girls. It didn't matter if dinner was waiting at home, if I wanted the taste of something extra, I just grabbed it in the privacy of my car and then, knowing it was wrong, I would destroy the evidence, or at least shove it under the seat. Nobody had to know.

Unfortunately for me, Irene was a wonderful detective or maybe I was just a sloppy binge eater. It didn't take her long to figure out the clues to my compulsive eating food addiction. Maybe it was the occasional hot sauce stains on my shirt, or the cream cheese on my cheek, or the fresh veggies left in a bag stuffed between the seats of our car. *I knew I should have just found a trash can!*

One look, and Irene could tell me how old the stain was or how long the veggies had been in hiding. Like a DEA agent at a drug bust, if she needed to "taste" the evidence on my clothes to confirm the offense, that's what she did. She usually didn't need to go that far. She was good and I wasn't getting away with anything. And even if I had, my increasing weight was proof positive that I was completely out of control.

It's very hard for me to watch old family videos of this time in our lives because it says everything without saying anything. We have one old video of me sprawled out in a recliner, trying to take a nap, while Amber is trying her best to get my attention. I slept through so much of their childhood, it's so sad. Call it the effects of raging sleep apnea or depression, or a mixture of both. Whatever it was, it was horrible. I was either eating, sleeping, or away at work. The times I was alert and actively pursuing quality time are the moments I hope they remember fondly. Too few, I'm sure. Courtney and Amber also remember the other side, the "be careful, don't wake the sleeping giant" side.

It wasn't easy carrying around the weight, trying to do everything a normal size person would do, but I adapted and managed as best I could. One trip to the Tulsa Zoo, I'll never forget. We walked the entire zoo, and I can't believe I survived. It was hot, I was sweating, and my weight made me miserable at best. The family video of the excursion shows that we took breaks regularly, but the most revealing moment of the video is the very last thing. While the girls visited the restroom by the exit, I focused the camera on the "Exit This Way" sign and then said out loud: *"It's over, thank God it's over."* This should have been a day that I *didn't* want to end, instead, I was enduring and simply surviving the nearly impossible task of moving under so much weight. I was looking forward to the air-conditioned comfort of my chair and another nap—after we eat, of course.

It was during this time in Tulsa that I tried the Atkins Diet. Everything about this plan sounded good to me. You mean I can eat all the bacon and cheese I want, and still lose weight? I've always been a meat and potatoes kind of guy, so now I decided I would become a meat and cheese kind of guy. This was easy. I bought the ketosis test strips and everything. I wanted to make sure the science was right. Then, I hit the grocery store. We spent about three times what we normally would have, buying loads of meat and eggs and several different kinds of cheese, and bacon! Dr. Atkins was a genius in my book. This was brilliant. Here was a diet that promised to drop the pounds without me ever confronting my food addict compulsive eating behaviors. I guess it all depends on how you approach this diet plan. I was approaching it with a fork and knife, licking my lips, and trading carbs for an eat-all-you-can meat buffet. I was ridiculously excited. I kept reading the part of the book about the science of it all, and proclaiming to Irene and anyone else that would listen, *"This guy has it all figured out, this is the answer!"* I was overjoyed—like an alcoholic discovering that they could drink a certain type of alcohol all they wanted, without any negative effects and without worrying about any of the unresolved problems and behaviors—that the addiction *smooths* over.

The first week, I was eating more food than I did before, and I was turning the test strip the appropriate color, signifying that I was in a state of ketosis. I started to lose weight right about the time I realized that I was getting sick of all the meat and cheese. I never realized how much I loved bread and sugar, and all things forbidden on the plan. I was seriously having a tough time, even on a plan that allowed me to gorge on pork skins and sharp cheddar all day. The biggest factor in me abandoning the plan was the expense. We simply couldn't afford the grocery bill. I guess I didn't give it a fair shot. But knowing what I know now and considering my food addict ways, any weight I could have lost would have been extremely temporary. I was glad to get that attempt out of my system, and now I could go another several months without giving weight loss a second thought.

As much as I tried to avoid it, I would think about losing weight again real soon. I could never really make it too long without something reminding me how serious my obesity was becoming. But my concern came in waves and then would go right back out with the tide of whatever circumstance we were enduring. Stress of any kind, owned me in every way. When life got tough (and thanks to our brilliant choices, it was mostly tough) I would eat. If emotions were getting the best of me, I would eat. Nervous, *eat*. Celebrating, *eat even more*. If I was using it as an escape, it was because it tasted *so good*. For the moments that it touched my lips and taste buds, I was in a state of joy, far, far away from the reality I was avoiding. If we were celebrating, I turned to food for the sheer pleasure of the experience. For someone so dependent on food, triggered by nearly every emotion imaginable, it's a real wonder I didn't eat myself to death.

I was very lucky to have so much love surrounding me, and that love, coupled with a career I felt comfortable doing, was enough to keep any depression over my size in check. In check, just enough, to continue doing whatever I wanted and continue being the giant of a man I had become. My family loved me and my colleagues respected me and my on-air abilities. I was talented for what I did, and without that element in my life, the constant reassurance of my worth to my family and my career, I'm not certain of my fate, considering my behaviors with food addiction.

I was on the air one Saturday afternoon when the phone line started flashing. It wasn't the usual request. The listener wanted me to come across the street to an oil company to talk to him about a radio station he was about to purchase. He wanted my opinion and after we met and talked for a short time, he wanted me to be his new program director and morning personality. What possesses an owner of a successful oil company to invest in a potential money pit of a small-market radio station? I'll never know. But, hey, we all have dreams. This was his dream. And after meeting me face to face, he wanted me to be a big part of his dream. I really liked this guy. I liked anyone who treated me so well, despite my morbid obesity. It's like he didn't even notice that I was so different. And that was an awesome thing. He wanted me for my experience and expertise, regardless of my appearance.

Forget that we were somewhat happy with our life in Tulsa, I was drawn to the flattery and acceptance. It was the first time someone was picking me out and offering me something I hadn't sought. It felt good to be wanted. It was like I was interviewing him and I would "let him know." He would be the one waiting by the phone, hoping I would say yes. I basked in this warm role reversal. He was offering a decent salary and told me to give him a figure that I needed for moving expenses. I said two thousand dollars, and he said "done," without any hesitation. The fact that the station he was buying was one I had worked for previously in Perry, Oklahoma, didn't seem to matter to me.

My enthusiasm for a return to Perry wasn't really shared by Irene, but we both agreed to make the move. After all, we would be closer to home. And the cost of living was cheaper and, really, if you get right down to the heart of the matter, I loved being wanted, being valued, being desired—all of it, despite my size. For someone who absolutely loathed himself ninety percent of the time, this was a huge step in the right direction of feeling better about who I was and what I could become.

Chapter Thirteen

Changes and Gravy

The new station was exciting. It was completely different from my previous experience in Perry. This time, the studios were brand new, and I was in charge of programming. Imagine that! I basically made it exactly like Star 103 in Tulsa, a 70's format, and we made a splash all over North Central Oklahoma. I was hitting my stride creatively on the morning show, and was even nominated for the Oklahoma Radio Personality of the Year award with the Oklahoma Association of Broadcasters. I was feeling great about myself career-wise, but physically, I was getting much worse.

My right leg was swelling to unnatural proportions because of the untreated lymphedema and I was still suffering with undiagnosed sleep apnea. I was good every day from about six AM to ten AM, then I was a complete wreck. The swelling would subside overnight and get worse as each day progressed. I had a tough time making it much past ten AM without dozing off uncontrollably. The owner of the station caught me sleeping during the last part of my show one morning and warned me that if he ever caught me doing that again, I was out. The fact that this was a medical issue wasn't discussed. I was falling asleep on the job and that was inexcusable. The occasional chest pain or shortness of breath brought on by the struggle to carry 500 pounds seemed to be the least of my concerns at that point. And the solution, in my mind, was always as simple as losing the weight. But still, I just couldn't wrangle my addiction. I couldn't stop being my own worst enemy. I was in extreme pain from my leg swelling and resulting sores, constantly tired, and occasionally would be convinced that I was dying of a heart attack, and still it *wasn't* enough to make me change.

I felt powerless to my addiction and the consequences. I was so lost and hopeless to my destructive compulsions. *But at least people loved hearing me on the radio!* I swear, my career and the love of family and friends kept me satisfied and hopeful that everything would be alright after-all. I could turn this all around with a determined plan. And that's exactly what I set out to do in October of 1996.

I decided that my time had come. *This was it.* This was going to be the time I actually lost the weight. I put together a simple plan that included eating a set amount of calories every day and walking at the new park walking trail in Perry. I made an arrangement with a professional photographer to take my picture every week for the duration of my transformation. I kept a notebook journal, much like my blog, and numbered each day. *It all sounds very familiar, I know.* But there was a critical difference.

I was teetering on disaster every day. I resented that I couldn't eat as much as I wanted. I hated limiting my portions, but I did it, because that's what I had to do to lose the weight. My focus wasn't on changing my behaviors with food. At that point, I hadn't really come to terms with the idea that I was a food addict. I just loved food, didn't everybody? I was super focused on the means to lose weight. Eat less and exercise more. *That's it.* I had no idea at the time that I was putting one hundred percent of my energy into twenty percent of the successful equation that I would later discover.

I was constantly looking forward to a cheat day. A day when I could forget all about this *eat less and exercise more nonsense*, and just be myself. It didn't dawn on me that my lust for food and losing control was a constantly present problem destined to derail me every time. A free day was a day that I could relax and just stuff myself in the name of freedom from the pressures and actions I needed to do to lose weight. I didn't want to hear about this being some kind of lifestyle change. *What? You mean I have to battle this for the rest of my life? Forget that!* I was temporarily changing my ways and looking forward to the perfect excuse to willingly jump off the wagon. Thanksgiving was coming up on day forty-something, and I couldn't think of a better day to cut loose. *I want extra gravy!*

In just over forty days, I had walked well over sixty miles around that same walking trail, I had visited the photographer five or six times and lost over forty pounds along the way. In my mind, I had earned a Thanksgiving free for all like no other. And I made sure the groceries were stocked for the occasion.

I had two pieces of pecan pie with whipped cream, first thing, for breakfast. This was going to be good. Thanksgiving dinner was planned at a hotel buffet with family. And I was determined to get my twelve bucks worth. I stuffed myself silly, probably making upwards of five trips to the buffet line, and knowing that more food was waiting at home.

A little rest, some antacids, and I'd be ready to go again later that evening. I was like a competitive eater in training. And the gravy tasted so good as it flowed over my tongue. The giant helping of mashed potatoes was ridiculous, but *dreamy* delicious. I refused to keep a calorie count that day. I didn't want to know and, honestly, I was eating so much so fast, I doubt I could have kept the tally accurate.

I justified this day because I had lost over forty pounds. I had worked hard and felt I deserved this day. I also convinced myself that it was only one day and really, *how much damage could one day create?* The answer to that question is actually two answers. Physically, maybe a pound or two of damage. Mentally, it was *complete destruction* of the groove I had created. The momentum was lost. That one day killed my drive completely. I tasted the gravy and never wanted to go back.

The next day was almost impossible to bear. I could feel it, this lost feeling. I felt completely out of control again. Even though that was yesterday, and this was today—a new day, time to get back on the horse. I just couldn't find the saddle or the desire to even look for the saddle. The horse I was riding for those forty-plus days of weight loss success was running free, far away from me, and what scared me the most was, I didn't seem to care.

I was embarrassed. I had even read my journal writings to some family and friends. They enjoyed the writing too and they were convinced that this was the time I would change it all. I would even drive by that park walking trail in Perry and think silently, *there it is, the trail where I'm finally walking off this obesity once and for all.*

Before Thanksgiving Day 1996, I was convinced and everyone around me was convinced that I was a seriously changed person. But after Thanksgiving, I was convinced that I was the same out-of-control compulsive eating food addict I'd always been. I didn't share this knowledge with anyone else, I just slowly reverted back to my old ways, and eventually everyone forgot about my latest failed attempt. I was seriously disappointed in myself. It didn't take long to gain back that forty-some pounds, plus some, and quickly, I was right back into a careless state of mind.

Chapter Fourteen

Becoming My Own Bully

Each time I would get serious about losing weight and then fail, it would take longer and longer to get back to the point of trying again. Instead of trying to lose weight, I was simply learning to accept myself as is, and that meant just dealing with the ailments that came with morbid obesity. I was successful at being a small-town radio personality, I had that. I was funny and, hey, wait a minute, *I was funny.* What if I made the best of my obesity and started doing stand-up comedy all about my size?

This was a brilliant plan really. I would follow my childhood dream of being a comedian, accepting the role as the fat guy, and audiences would give me love in return for being me, all 500 pounds of me. *Who needs to lose weight?* Heck, it might become my trademark! If enough people laughed and thought I was funny, maybe I could be convinced to love my size. I needed my size to start earning a paycheck in order for me to justify my inaction toward trying to do anything to lose the weight and become healthier.

It was a *meant to be moment,* when I decided to call the comedy clubs in Oklahoma City and Tulsa on a Tuesday, and to my surprise, they both had a scheduled open-mic for that night. What's even more *meant to be-ish,* is the time I called Tulsa. It was ten AM. I had no idea that this was the time new comics were instructed to call for a spot on Tuesday nights. I accidentally called my way into a five-minute set scheduled for ten hours after making the initial call. Yeah, *this was meant to be.* But I needed some jokes. I quickly hurried home from work and recruited Irene to help me write my first five-minute set.

My first line, *"I weigh three hundred and ninety-eight pounds,"* was a flat out lie. But so was the idea that I enjoyed making fun of myself on stage. I decided it didn't have to be true, just funny. And I knew I had the presentation skills to pull it off. Besides, I never appeared to be 500 pounds. When people would try to guess my weight, they most usually would guess seventy-five to a hundred pounds less than I actually weighed. And I was too embarrassed to say my real weight in front of anyone. Three hundred and ninety-eight sounded funny to me, for some strange reason. Like I was very mindful of *not hitting* 400 pounds, or something.

I went straight for the bottom of the barrel stuff. *"When you see a person my size, the first question that normally comes to mind is, how do they have sex? Well, I'm here to tell you . . . alone."* It isn't really funny on paper, but with the delivery I gave, it killed. My closer was a rap parody of the Vanilla Ice song Ice Ice Baby. Irene and I wrote it in about thirty minutes and we were so proud. This was comedy genius: *"Alright, stop, collaborate and listen. Sean is back with my brand new addiction, food, grabs a hold of me tightly, I roll like a big whale daily and nightly. Will I ever stop, yo, I just grow, bring out the food, and I'll go—to the extreme, stopping short of a cannibal, open the fridge and watch me eat like an animal. OBESE, with a belly that shakes, I'm killing LA with the ten point earthquakes, DEADLY, when I eat the way I do, because sometimes I forget to chew. Eat it, don't leave it, you better gain weight, you better eat it all, cause the kid don't play. If there is food then, yo, I'll eat it, check out your plate while my hand retrieves it."* Of course, the rap was accompanied by my best 500-pound, *uh, I mean,* 398-pound dance moves, simply to punctuate the funny. And believe it or not, it worked like a charm.

The reaction from the audience after my first set was intoxicating. I felt at home on stage, even being nervous, it just added to my appeal with these drunk comedy club patrons. I walked into the bar area and everyone was congratulating me on my set. *I had made an impression.* The biggest compliment was from the bar tender, an aspiring comic himself. He said, *"I got chills watching you, you're going to be amazing."* This was all I needed to hear. I was hooked completely. As my material evolved and eventually included me dropping the rap, it still was all about my size, and I was still pretending to be a hundred pounds lighter than I actually was, the compliments kept coming from several people, independent of each other. I kept hearing things that overjoyed me, like the whole *"gave me chills"* line, over and over. And when an established comedian told me I had the "it" factor. Oh, my, my addiction to self-deprecating stand-up comedy turned into an all-out obsession. I wanted to get better and better, and the only way to do that was to get as much stage time as possible, every chance I possibly could.

Finally, I had found a way to accept and thrive in my obesity. Losing weight was the furthest thing from my mind at this point. The addiction to love and acceptance I found on stage led me to do some pretty drastic things. Even if we were broke, I would find a way to get to Tulsa or Oklahoma City to perform. If it meant taking our last twenty bucks, I did it. *Why?* Because I was pursuing us a better life, of course. *This was the sacrifice part.* The reward part would come later, just be patient, was what I told Irene and the girls, over and over. It will all pay off someday, you just wait and see, *I have the "it" factor, by golly!* I was destined for comedy stardom and nobody could convince me otherwise.

It didn't take long for me to start getting paid gigs as an opening act. The money was far less than I imagined it would be. Often times, two hundred bucks or less for the entire Wednesday through Sunday run of shows. If the club was in Oklahoma City or Tulsa, then I would drive every night, eating away at the money. But I wasn't doing it for the money, *damn it,* I was doing it for the experience. Bigger things were coming my way, this was just training.

My first big gig came eight months into my young stand-up career. I somehow conned the student organizers of Oklahoma State's Orange Peel into letting me be the opening act for Faith Hill and Sinbad. I would also be the "Voice of the Peel." I quickly rushed out and paid two hundred dollars for a seamstress to measure, design, and create a custom-fit bright orange sport coat. The custom tailored jacket with a black gangster looking hat completed my giant orange look for this stadium gig in front of twenty-six thousand people. I was *so not ready* for this gig. The voice work, sure—I had ten years plus experience in voice-overs and broadcasting; the comedy—no, *I wasn't ready.* But you couldn't have convinced me of the truth. I was blinded by my passion and fueled by the compliments of my comedy buddies around me. I was destined for greatness in the comedy world, and this gig was a sure sign of that future. *Or so I thought.*

The gig was a disaster in so many ways. My set was ten minutes long, but I knew violent storms were headed straight for the stadium. And since I had called the National Weather Service media line before I went on stage, I knew the storms would probably arrive before I finished my set. The first part of my set wasn't going well. The atmosphere in this open air stadium was a million miles from an enclosed and intimate comedy club. I heard some faint laughter from the thousands in attendance, but mainly I just heard things like, *"you suck!"* and *"get off the stage!"*

I was quickly sinking and then the worst of it started. Lightning and thunder roared over a stadium full of metal seats and thousands of people sitting up high. *This wasn't good.* And since I was also the voice of the event, the director came out right before my big closer and tried to communicate an urgent message.

At first, I wasn't stopping. I was trucking along, no matter how many *"you sucks"* I heard. But when the director of the show came on stage in the middle of a now, driving thunderstorm, I knew I had to stop. The storm was so loud, I could barely hear what he was screaming. It was like that scene in *Back to the Future*, when Doc

Brown is trying to get Marty back to 1995, and right there in the middle of the storm, Marty is trying to tell Doc about the terrorist. *"You must read this to the crowd."* I need to do what? *"You need to read this weather report to the crowd, immediately."* The rain was loud, punctuated with loud strikes of lightening as thousands ran for cover. I swear, even during this crazy moment, I thought to myself, *this couldn't wait until my big finish?*

"Ladies and gentlemen, the National Weather Service has issued a severe thunderstorm warning for Payne County. This storm contains frequent lightening and the possibility of hail. The show will continue, but please stay at your own risk." Or something to that effect. Right after I finished that official statement, the director told me to introduce Sinbad right then and there. I was flustered from the storm and the fact that I didn't get to finish my set. Sinbad came out and did six minutes of material on how crazy it was to be performing in the middle of a violent thunderstorm. The storm became severe and the show had to be canceled and I, along with Sinbad, was taken to the safety and shelter of the stadium press box. Faith Hill never left the comfort and safety of her hotel room, Sinbad did six minutes, and I did nearly ten minutes. The show was canceled and twenty-six thousand people were not happy. I swear, I thought each and every one in that stadium hated me, except my family and friends, of course.

The after-party included Sinbad hanging out and chatting with everyone involved. He felt horrible about the turn of events, and since he was being paid fifty thousand dollars, he agreed to come back and do a show whenever they could re-schedule. Talking to Sinbad and hearing his account of his rise to fame in the comedy world just fueled my desire even more. I was inspired to charge forward, even if a large crowd was chanting *"you suck,"* just a couple of hours before. In my mind, I didn't suck (I did), I just wasn't as funny as Sinbad or as attractive as Faith Hill, that's all.

My stock in the comedy world was on the rise. I could now honestly proclaim that I had opened for Sinbad and Faith Hill, and that must mean I was good enough to be an opener for one-seventy-five a week. Eventually, my insane quest to pay my dues in the world of comedy caught up to my marriage. I was booked for a week at the Looney Bin Comedy Club in Wichita when I learned that Irene and I were separating.

It was a blow to me, but strangely, not enough for me to see my contribution to the unfolding destruction of our family. I hurried home from that gig and realized that things were changing beyond my control. Instead of making me want to change my direction, it simply sent me into a constant state of depression and pleading for her and the girls to come back. I still wasn't doing anything about my weight and I was still driving all over the Southwest doing comedy gigs for next to nothing, while trying to maintain my job in radio. And I did it all, while suffering from the horrible effects of sleep apnea. That was the kicker for Irene. I could somehow manage to make it all over the place for comedy gigs, but before the comedy obsession, it was eat, sleep, work, and sleep some more.

Chapter Fifteen

Losing Everything But Weight

I was swerving along the highway one night, on my way home from the Tulsa Comedy Club, fighting sleep all the way, when a trooper pulled me over and ordered me to nap on the side of the road. I gave him my home number and he called Irene to tell her of my roadside slumber. For the few seconds it took the trooper to explain, Irene was convinced that I was in a horrible accident. I was paying my comedy dues, that's all. Never mind that my young family was falling apart. The end would justify the means, *if* the end included an insanely successful comedy career. It was just a gamble that took its toll on everyone around me. Eventually, after falling asleep in a hotel room in Elk City, exhausted after a comedy one-nighter, and missing my morning show the next day, I lost my radio job. I was quickly approaching rock bottom. I had lost my family, my job, and I honestly felt like I was losing my mind and health, all in a blind pursuit of something that made me feel so good about myself, *while destroying me piece by piece.*

Somehow, someway, I eventually convinced the broadcasting company that fired me to re-hire me at their Ponca City studios. I was still separated from Irene and the girls, so I would be moving to Ponca City on my own. I was still pursuing comedy, though not as much as before. It was something I just couldn't shake. I just knew that big things were in my future, I couldn't give up now.

I settled into a routine that included the radio show, doing as many comedy sets as I possibly could in Tulsa and Oklahoma City, and every now and then, begging Irene to come back with the girls. When it seemed hopeless that we would ever get back together, I started dating a few different people. That's right—fueled by the confidence that the stage gave me, I found a way to overcome my 500 pounds of insecurities and actually date. Those were all short-lived relationships. One ended abruptly when the girl asked me what I really wanted and I told her that all I really wanted was my wife and kids back. Yeah, that was a mood killer apparently. At least I was honest about what I wanted, you have to give me that.

As my desire for the return of my family grew, and I wasn't getting what I really wanted, I poured myself into radio and stand-up. Radio kept me going financially and comedy was like a drug habit I just couldn't let go. I lived for the natural high of making a packed comedy club erupt in laughter. If I wasn't working or doing a comedy gig, I was with my daughters, spending time, always punctuated with me pleading with Irene for the reassembly of our family unit. It was a tiresome routine that kept me from getting too depressed. As long as I kept getting paid from KLOR, I would survive. As long as the comedy club audiences kept laughing, I would keep getting stage time. And as long as Irene was still listening to my desperate pleas, I would keep talking, and hoping for a reunion. This was my life.

Losing weight was the furthest thing from my mind. I was obsessed with everything *but my weight.* Eventually, Irene became tired of my relentless begging. She had enough of me the first time. I couldn't blame her really. When she applied for a restraining order to keep me away, I was crushed and completely broken. The order was denied by the judge because I wasn't physically abusive, I was just annoyingly persistent. Good thing they don't hand out restraining orders against people that are *just annoying,* because if they did, they would need an entire separate court system to handle the requests. Irene wasn't happy and I wasn't either. And my daughters were lovingly surviving through it all. It was a painful time that was about to become much worse because of a totally unrelated tragic turn of events.

Section Three

California Dreaming

"My quest for acceptance and love takes me to the brink of comedy success, before I realize, the joke is on me."

Chapter Sixteen

Shane's Gift

I spent the night with Mom and Shane on June 16th, 2001. I slept on their couch that night. Shane wasn't feeling well and had voiced that he had decided to stay home from work the next day. I wish I would have stayed home with him that day, but there wasn't any reason to believe that life wouldn't just go on like normal. It was a normal day, until I answered my cell phone and Kelli, obviously upset, informed me that Shane had been rushed to the emergency room in Stillwater. This wasn't a minor situation and I needed to be there. I flew down US Highway 177 as fast as I could, trying to reassure myself that everything was going to be alright with Shane. My internal hope mechanism just couldn't forget the urgency I heard in Kelli's voice. Shane had to survive whatever this was, *because we had plans, damn it.* We needed time.

I was looking forward to continuing the growth of our relationship. If my teenage romance, eventual marriage, and developing family kept me away from Shane, I was now looking forward to making up for lost time. I loved taking Shane to the comedy clubs. It made him feel so good to be sitting in the back with the comics. He was with me, and everyone that met my little brother knew how special he was to me and everyone else. Shane looked up to me in so many ways. In his eyes I could do no wrong. His forgiving heart excused me from years of brotherly neglect while I hit the fast forward button on life in an ignorant attempt to grow up too fast.

I wanted to take Shane and show him the world. I wanted him to experience everything he thought impossible for someone with his mental handicap. You see, Shane may have been mildly mentally challenged, but he still had the capacity to dream and inspire, spreading his love unconditionally, while being acutely aware of the limitations society reserved for him. It was those unfair restrictions that frustrated Shane to no end. *What a cruel level of impairment,* I thought. To have the ability to dream and desire, with the mental capacity to understand that these were things he was never expected to accomplish. Like driving a car, or experiencing the intimacy of a kiss, or performing on stage like his big brother. All of these things, I had hoped to introduce to him in time, but on that day, the changes and plans were not of mine or anyone's desire.

I rushed into the emergency room and was immediately greeted with the sobering shock of an unspeakable feeling that was confirming our worst fears. Everyone was gathered in the emergency room waiting area while the doctors and nurses tried everything they knew how to save my brother's life. Shane had become sick in his sleep. When he coughed, he ended up vomiting, and in his half-asleep state, he inhaled the waste into his lungs. He had aspirated. And saving his life at this point wasn't going to be easy.

The doctor eventually came out and gave us an assessment of the situation. The doctor's body language communicated a grim reality I didn't want to accept. He informed us that Shane was basically dead on arrival. His team had successfully resuscitated him and he was stabilized, but only with the assistance of machines that were keeping him alive. I knew what this meant, I think we all did. *What happens if the machines are turned off? Was there any hope for recovery?* We were given a sliver of hope that Shane would survive as they wheeled him and the machines that were keeping him alive up to the intensive care unit.

Irene showed up quickly, offering support, and grieving alongside all of us. The dynamic of our family unit may have been in shambles, but we were all brought together that day, in love and sadness for my fallen brother. Our marital differences were put aside completely as we endured this tragedy, leaning on each other to cope. Suddenly, our issues seemed small in comparison to the bigger picture. Our plans seemed so pointless and out of reach, but it didn't matter. Every ounce of our energy was being offered up in prayers that Shane would somehow survive. *If only you will give Shane another chance, he has so much left to do, he's only twenty-four, please don't take him,* I'd pray. And honestly, I was praying for my *second chance* to be the brother he deserved.

I thought I had all the time in the world with Shane. Someday we were going to do everything we dreamed of doing, but *someday* never came up on the calendar before June 19th, 2001, the day he died. I'll never forget standing outside of his ICU room with my arm around my mom, who was in a constant state of shock, and watching as the heart monitor slowed and then stopped, completely flat. This wasn't supposed to happen. I wasn't ready to let him go, none of us were. Suddenly, the someday that Shane and I dreamed of became feelings of sorrow over the regretful procrastination of the life we craved. It was a lesson that I would eventually analyze, learn from, and benefit from as my weight loss philosophy and resolve developed along the way. It was a lesson in doing things today, instead of an undetermined and *uncertain someday.* It was the basis for the simplistic idea of choosing change *before change chooses me.*

Shane wanted to do everything I could. So how dare I waste the opportunity to live up to my potential, when Shane would have given anything to experience a fraction of what I mostly took for granted. This was a turning point for me. Shane's tragic death lit a fire within me, a more determined spirit than ever before, to see my dreams become reality.

My brother also gave me hope, taught me things, and gave me and everyone around him a renewed and thorough understanding of compassion and love. It's no wonder why he received the biggest ovation of anyone at his high school graduation. It was even bigger than the one reserved for the biggest star athlete in the class, Matt Holliday, who would go on to become a Major League All-Star slugger.

Shane touched lives in that school. His performance of Garth Brooks's The River, accompanied on guitar by his fellow classmate and future recording artist Stoney Larue at the high school talent show, left everyone in attendance changed. The special education teachers immediately noticed a rise in students applying to become peer advocates in the special needs classroom. Shane was inspiring change with his beautiful song, far beyond what he could have ever imagined. And he inspired me, and still does to this day, in everything I do *and dream.* He'll always be with me. *Always.*

Chapter Seventeen

U-Turns

The wave of weight-related concern would come again and leave me scrambling for some kind of plan. I had tried so many things, from simply counting calories to Nutri-System, the Atkins Diet, and my own counting calories, walking, and journaling plan, complete with the weekly picture by a professional photographer. Still, something vitally important was missing from every previous attempt.

I decided to try my own brand of the Atkins plan combined with calorie counting. This new "plan" accomplished very little, besides entertaining my co-workers at the Team Radio studios. My plan included eating pork rinds, Vienna sausages, and cheese every day at lunch. This combination of foods was going to change my life! Bill, Jerry, Gayle, and Ryan took it all in and immediately recognized the absurdity of it all. I didn't understand why they were laughing. This wasn't funny, by golly, this was the plan! I can laugh about it now, and yes, it still occasionally comes up for comic relief around the Team Radio studios, but for about a week, I really thought I had found the answer. I still love an occasional pork rind or Vienna sausage, but poor calorie values have excluded these from becoming a regular part of my dietary intake. That's probably a good thing.

I carried a temporary air about me during this time in my life. In my mind, everything was temporary, my commitment to radio was just waiting for my stand-up career to blossom, and my living single and casual dating experiences were just waiting to come to a joyous end with an embrace and reunion with Irene and the girls. When a remote broadcast fell on the same day as one of my pre-booked comedy gigs, I learned that my determined nature had nothing on the dog-gone-it-all stubbornness of one, Mr. Jerry Vaughn, the operations manager and my boss at Team Radio.

In fairness to me, the gig was a private corporate gig, booked far in advance of this remote broadcast. But in fairness to Jerry, he had let me "off the hook" many times. And since I completely wrecked a broadcast with an oil spill slowly progressing toward a crowd of one hundred just a few days prior, Jerry wasn't in the mood to budge.

It's an ironic story. The remote broadcast I wrecked was Dave May's final weigh-in after completing exactly one year on the Subway Diet and losing 111 pounds. Dave raised over one hundred thousand dollars with this effort, enough to help build a new youth services shelter.

I didn't mean to wreck the broadcast. I had checked the oil in the remote vehicle generator and didn't quite get the lid back on straight. Oil shot out of the motor in frightening amounts, slowly making its way toward the gathered crowd surrounding the scale on the sidewalk in front of the downtown Subway Sandwich Shop. I was focused on cleaning up the spill and totally missed my cue at exactly 12:30 PM. I had left Jerry live, hanging on the air, scrambling for words, without this monumental weigh-in report. The report was a year in the making. Jerry was totally unforgiving.

If I wanted to save my job, I had to cancel this stand-up gig, forfeiting the five-hundred-dollar fee for thirty minutes work. Any reasonable individual would have reluctantly found another comic to take his place, choosing instead to maintain good graces at the place that keeps the lights on. I wasn't being reasonable, or mature, or professional for that matter.

I decided to resign my position with Team Radio with an infamous resignation letter that named names and would become legendary in the halls of Team Radio. Jerry and Gayle, according to the letter, *"the two most negative people I have ever known,"* had the letter changed to calligraphy and then posted it prominently in the KLOR studio for all to see. It was waiting for me when I returned to Team Radio for the fourth time and it remained on the wall for several years. Yes, *a fourth time,* but I'm getting ahead of myself.

I wasn't canceling my corporate stand-up gig, even if it meant losing my job with Team Radio. But before you think I'm crazy, I did have a back-up plan. In my back pocket was a job offer from a new station sixty miles away, a new station that promised complete flexibility with my stand-up schedule. A new station that was so new, they hadn't even decided what to call themselves, let alone, how to program the station. This was an opportunity for me to brand this station from the very beginning. This station wasn't your average commercial grade FM powerhouse. In fact, it wasn't even licensed as a commercial station. It was a low power FM signal. This was a few notches above pirate radio, but I didn't care, as long as the paychecks kept coming and nobody complained when I left early on a Thursday for a weekend stand-up gig at the Amarillo Comedy Club.

My first clue that things were not good, and maybe I was crazy after all, came when the FCC walked in flashing badges and proceeded to shut us down. I'm thinking: no signal, no programming, no job, all adds up to *no paycheck.* But it was a false alarm. We just waited until the FCC inspector left the building, then we turned it back on. I swear, *we didn't wait until he left town.* We were pirates, arrrgh!

The second clue came when I took my paycheck to the bank and the tellers gathered around and proceeded to laugh at me. I wish I was exaggerating for the sake of comedy. I'm not. The teller took one look at the check and busted up. Her reaction attracted other bank employees, who must have just had a meeting about this very account, because they joined in the laughter. *I wasn't laughing.* I was broke and this was my paycheck to make me not broke. Instead it made me embarrassed and mostly regretful that I blazed my way out of Team

Radio on a burning bridge. I didn't need a third clue to conclude that I was in trouble. Yes, sir, I was in a real bad situation that was probably going to require me to swallow my pride, prepare an apology, and practically beg my way across that charred bridge. Lucky for me, good Ole Jer had a sense of humor. Not lucky for me was my timing.

"Hello, Jerry. Hey, it's Sean. Sean Anderson! Listen, uh, I think I owe you, Gayle, and Bill a big apology. Jerry? Jerry? Did I catch you at a bad time? Oh, you were busy being negative about something, I see. Jerry, I've made a horrible mistake. Yes, I think you're, uh, Jerry, please, if you just give me a chance to redeem myself, I swear, I'll make it up to you. You know the kind of work I'm capable of doing. Oh, well, thank you, Jerry, thank you for saying that. But you've, uh, you've hired someone new just yesterday you say? Wow, horrible timing, huh? It was good talking with you, Jerry, thank you for taking my call." As soon as we hung up, I knew exactly what took place in his office. Everyone hit the floor laughing hysterically at this horrible turn of events. I deserved it really. Honestly, I did.

I had left myself in a really bad position. Since the new job situation turned out the way it did, I qualified for unemployment. And it wasn't long before Team Radio called offering me a way to get my foot back in the door, with an offer of a part-time job on their sports talk station. It was something to help supplement the sporadic stand-up gig revenue. The stress of it all kept me a million miles away from even thinking about losing weight. I had other worries, like how to pay my bills and what about getting my family back together?

My separation from Irene was quickly approaching two years when we finally agreed that we should give it all another try. Neither one of us wanted a divorce, obviously, so resuming our married life would be fairly simple. We both contributed issues to the demise of our marriage in the first place, and we both knew that if we were putting it back together, then we needed a new understanding.

My part of the deal included being a little more picky about what stand-up gigs I accepted. I was no longer driving horribly long distances just to get stage time. If I wasn't getting paid, I wasn't doing the gig. That made a big difference. I still had the dream alive inside me, that same dream that compelled me on numerous occasions to drive clear across the state on little sleep, for no money and five minutes on a Dallas stage. Yeah, I did that on several occasions. But never again. Unless, that stage time in Dallas meant auditioning for CBS and the New Star Search!

Chapter Eighteen

Star Scorch

There was a large community of stand-up comics online and I was constantly on the message boards. We all kept in touch, made fun of each other, and stayed up to date on the goings on in our industry. When the new Star Search announced auditions for comics in Dallas, I immediately decided, I was going. *This was my shot. This was it,* and after a short conversation, Irene and the girls gave me their blessing. They knew that I was dreaming of finally giving them the better life I had always promised. They believed in me.

It was time to put on a smile and play the part of the funny fat guy. Deep down, I hated the "character" I had created in my stand-up routine. But I had learned a long time before to just keep them laughing. If they were laughing, that meant they loved me. And if they loved me, *what could I complain about?* Never mind that it wasn't truly the real me; the real *me* would never treat myself with so much disregard.

Billy Gardell, now the star of CBS's "Mike and Molly," once told me that if I ever figured out how much the audience liked me, it would be like turning a key. I think I was finally understanding what he meant. *I could have just been myself,* instead of this very believable character. The audiences would have liked me even more . . . *like turning a key.*

What possessed me to constantly bully myself for the sake of comedy? It was my way of avoiding the issue of food addiction and compulsive eating by embracing, almost celebrating, my morbid obesity. It was horribly self-deprecating, and it was sadly, self-accepting. I was giving up on ever losing the weight. Not really, I mean, in the back of my mind I would always think, *someday.* And if a loved one expressed concern and worry for my health, I would of course, assure them that I would be doing something about it, uh, *very soon.* Yeah, *just relax, it's going to be OK,* I'll worry about that real soon. *Just not right now.* I had a national TV show waiting for me to audition!

Actually, they weren't waiting for me yet, but I was coming. I was headed to Big D with my best two minutes ready to go. My Aunt Kelli and my comedy buddy Cruz Carr accompanied me as we embarked on what could have been our big break.

The Star Search talent coordinators divided us into groups of about twenty and sent us into these big rooms. They would call each of our names and when you heard your name, you walked forward to the center of the room and immediately delivered your best two minutes. My nerves were flipping out. *This was go time.* I'm surprised I even heard my name called because I was too busy going over my tried and true two minutes of guaranteed funny. *Scene Anderson, you're up.* Uh, that's Sean Anderson, like Sean Connery or Sean Penn. *Great, the first words out of my mouth and I'm correcting the talent scouts. I hope that doesn't count toward my two minutes.* I recovered nicely and dived right into a familiar flow and groove that I had hit out of the park so many times on comedy club stages. *They were laughing, they're laughing!!! Stay cool, stay cool, finish strong, finish strong.* I was on total auto-pilot. My mouth was delivering the material but my mind was analyzing their reactions by the millisecond.

When my two minutes worth had expired, perfectly punctuated with a well-paced and perfectly delivered closer, they laughed and then called out another name. *Chad Dubrul, you're up. Oh, my, if I'm competing against Chad, I might as well go home,* I thought. Chad was easily one of the funniest guys I had ever worked with. His prerecorded opener while eating a Snickers Bar was absolutely brilliant. He was drop dead funny, seriously experienced, and he was killing with the candy bar, again, and again. *It always worked.* And I wondered if he would toss me the leftover candy bar like he did when we worked together in Tulsa. *That would be hysterical. If he does, I'm devouring it right then and there, that would be over-the-top hilarious.*

He didn't toss me the candy and that was just fine, because within minutes, Chad and I were asked to stay behind along with a couple of others. The rest were dismissed, never to return. We were given a little break and then asked to perform again for the same two talent coordinators. This was the second call back. Again, the nerves, the set . . . oh, my, I just used my best two minutes, now what? I had thirty or so more minutes to choose from, but nothing like the Subway diet bit! I picked something, I honestly can't remember what, and it was time to wait for the phone to ring.

All of us second call-back comics were asked to stay in the area and wait for a phone call. If we didn't receive a call, we didn't make it. If we did get a call, then we were coming back the next day for another round of auditions. My friend Cruz didn't pass, and he really needed to get back home to Norman, so we decided to stay overnight in a Norman motel. Kelli and I talked about Star Search all the way to Norman. We grew up watching the original, every episode. It was crazy that now, I was on the brink of being on the show, at least it felt that way.

I excitedly called home and shared the news. Irene and the girls were so happy and my mom and everyone else were overjoyed with excitement. Waiting for that phone call and realizing that it might not come, was complete torture. I must have stared at that phone for two hours straight, trying to will it to ring. And finally, at almost nine PM, it did. *"Hey, Sean, JP Buck with Star Search. We really enjoyed your material today and we would love you to come back tomorrow and give us some more."* I was beside myself happy. I barely hung up from the call when tears of joy started streaming down my face. Kelli was getting emotional, too. We were witnessing my dream come true. *They liked me, they really liked me.* All of a sudden, the improbable seemed completely possible. I quickly made another round of calls to share the latest good news. We were headed back to Dallas the next morning where I would audition for the third time on very little sleep. Oh, I had all night to sleep, but my mind wouldn't shut off. Like a kid trying to sleep before a big vacation trip, I was too excited. I just laid there looking up at the ceiling, dreaming all night with my eyes wide open.

The call-back was scheduled for ten AM. I walked into the lobby and immediately discovered what one of my fellow comics thought of me. His shocked reaction said it all. *YOU made it, too?* I had no idea that he doubted my talent. He always pretended to like me, but he certainly revealed himself with his puzzled query. It didn't matter. I was minutes away from my audition and I couldn't be bothered with his negative emotions. I walked into a private audition this time and after nailing another three-minute set, the talent scouts pulled me aside. They told me that they really enjoyed my stuff and they wanted me to come back in a few hours for one last audition. This time in front of the network people and every segment producer on the show. This big audition in front of a panel of twelve was a hush-hush thing. I was warned: "Don't tell anyone else about this because only a couple out of everyone we've auditioned in Dallas will get to do it, and you're one of them. Just relax for a few hours and come back this afternoon ready to go into the big room."

Kelli was across the street at Denny's waiting for me to finish. I was a nervous wreck as I walked across the parking lot toward Denny's. I felt a high like I had never known. It was a confidence that completely overpowered any insecurity my 500-pound body tried to create. I walked into the restaurant and told Kelli the amazing news. There was a group of comics I didn't know sitting at a table across the way, so I had to be quiet, whispering, *because this was a super secret call-back.* I was in exclusive company. There were comics that were far more experienced than me and in my opinion, much funnier than me, who had been rejected. My confidence was strong as I chalked it up to what people had said to me, you know, about the "it" factor. Yeah, it had to be the "it."

It's a very strange feeling to be so confident, yet so scared at the same time. When the lunch crowd started thinning, I was able to open up more with Kelli about what I was feeling. I was overwhelmed with emotions. I had always been a dreamer, but never did I feel this close to having one of my dreams actually come true. I kept thinking about all we had been through over the years. I thought about Shane and how he would be so proud of me, and actually, he would have been on that trip, *I'm sure.*

I thought about my daughters and Irene and the life I always dreamed of giving them. I wanted to make my momma cry tears of joy, *I did. Could my talent take me there? To the place where dreams really do come true?* All those nights traveling down the highway, fighting sleep, and just trying to get to the next stage. Paying dues that far exceeding the pennies I would earn, *finally,* it was all going to pay off. I would be on that show. I would win and it would completely change the course of our future.

Before long it was nearly time to walk back across the parking lot and perform for the panel of Star Search producers and CBS entertainment executives. JP Buck greeted me in the lobby and asked how I was doing. He told me to breathe and I thanked him for reminding me. We walked toward some big double doors of a ballroom and stopped just short of stepping inside. I thought I had a few minutes to get ready, but no, that was what the last three hours was for. JP quickly told me that he would open the door and lead me into the room. He would introduce me as I walked straight to the microphone to immediately start my material. JP asked if I understood. *Uh, yeah, yeah, I understand.* And like someone being pushed into the water and told to sink or swim, the door flew open and JP quickly walked into the room introducing me. I went straight to the microphone and proceeded to do my best five minutes. I made the panel laugh right away as I fought the urge to go into auto-pilot again, letting my mind wander around the room and the faces before me. I had to focus, and I did just that.

I felt great about the performance and then they asked me to stick around for some direct questions from the panel. JP didn't mention this part. Maybe he didn't know they would want to ask questions. I couldn't decide if this was a good thing or not, but either way, I didn't have time to think. The first question was about where I grew up. I told them a little about Stillwater and my neighborhood. The second question was about my family. I wasn't expecting this and I wasn't emotionally ready to talk about how much I loved them and wanted to do well for them. I started to lose it, my voice was quivering, and then, after I had mentioned my wonderful momma, a panelist asked me: *"How's your relationship with your father?"*

At this point, my lips were trembling, too, and the tears started streaming down my face. It took everything I had to hold back a full-fledged sobbing. "I never knew my father. He left before I was born." *Why, why, why? Why did they have to go there? And why couldn't I just put on a smile and pretend everything was fine?* I was an emotional wreck. I tried to explain my emotions by saying that I was just happy to be there, but I'm afraid I came off as emotionally unstable. You know those people who cry when they make it to Hollywood on American Idol? It was those kind of tears. Surely, these tears of joyful redemption wouldn't be held against me.

On the other side of the door, JP assured me that I did great and told me that they would start making the final decisions closer to Thanksgiving and taping was to start the first part of January in Los Angeles. I had done everything I could do at that point. And even though I had an uneasy feeling about my emotional display, I still made the drive back to Stillwater with the confidence that I would make it on the show. It was just a matter of waiting for the final word.

It wasn't two weeks later when I checked my voice mail and found a message from JP Buck. *"Sean, JP Buck from Star Search, give me a call.* " I played that message over and over. It gave me chills. I knew that this was the call. I had made it on the show. They didn't call to tell you *you* didn't make it. If I hadn't made it on, they would have just lost my number and forgotten about me. I had a nervous excitement that was teetering on euphoria while I dialed his number. When he answered, it wasn't what I was hoping to hear. *"We need you to send us a tape of you in a comedy club, doing different material, preferably non-weight-related stuff. Maybe do some family-type material. We're still deciding. Just send the tape and we'll go from there."*

Now what? My best material was spent *and* my best material was weight related. I was about to panic when I decided to pull it together and make it happen. I called Randy, the manager-owner of the Tulsa Comedy Club and explained the situation to him. Randy was a big supporter and quickly offered a Saturday night guest set. I called everyone I knew to invite them to this big show. I needed a huge audience, stacked in my favor. This tape was a one-shot deal and I wasn't taking any chances. I even called my broadcast colleagues at KRMG and explained the Star Search story in hopes of getting an interview on the most listened to news-talk station in town. I was creating a buzz about the show. They quickly agreed to have me on during afternoon drive with Denver Fox. The family and friends were invited and now all I needed was some new material. This was a very backward way of doing things, but not unlike many of the things in my life.

The idea of writing fresh and completely unproven material, then debuting that material on a Saturday night before a packed comedy club, with the camera rolling on a tape to be sent to CBS, is absolutely insane. But this was the plan. They wanted a tape and I had come too far to throw in the towel now.

I immediately started writing material based on getting married at seventeen years old and having kids way too young. *"We didn't have a wedding reception, we had a pep rally."* And *"we saved a bunch of money on the honeymoon because at the Holiday Inn, kids stay for free."* Oh, and . . . *"A friend of mine suggested we sign a prenuptial agreement. To protect what? My bicycle? Baby, if this don't work out, you ain't gettin' my Huffy. I threw newspapers to get that."*

I explored the rules of parenthood too: *"When your kid draws you a picture, you are required to keep it forever. We were at a friend's house the other night and my daughter drew the most beautiful picture on their front door. And I said, well, my friend, it looks like I'm gonna have to take your door home and put it on my refrigerator."* It wasn't the strongest material ever written, but I was convinced that I had the personality to pull it off. The show was a few days away and the only test of this new stuff was delivering it over a game of cards and drinks with Irene and my cousin Candi and her husband Tim. The three of them thought the new stuff was strong. But so were the drinks that night, maybe that helped the funny. The comedy club crowd would be drinking, too, but I knew the powers at Star Search would more than likely be sober. The material needed to carry, regardless.

I was so upset with myself because I had performed countless shows without ever writing too much new non-weight-related material. Oh, I had some, but the meat and potatoes of my set was always dependent on my size. It was pure laziness. A complete lack of preparation for this moment. What do they say about luck being *preparation meeting opportunity?* Yeah, *that.* I had positioned myself on the opposite side of luck, and I knew that it would take a miracle to pull it all together.

If you invite a hundred people and twenty show up, you're doing good. The crowd was smaller than I had hoped for, much smaller than a typical Saturday night Tulsa show, but I didn't have time to worry about the crowd size. The tape was rolling and I had ten minutes to hit it out of the park. The pressure was horrible. Every second was being captured and as much as I tried to forget, I knew that it would eventually be viewed by the people in LA. I was trying way too hard and when the first big punch kind of fizzled, I felt like I was going to die. There were no do-overs. I wasn't having this video edited; they would surely frown on that. So I just kept going and somehow managed a respectable set. It wasn't the over-the-top performance I had hoped to capture, but it was me, delivering non-weight-related material in a comedy club setting, just as Star Search requested.

I couldn't get to the post office fast enough on Monday morning. I paid the extra money for overnight delivery and by Tuesday morning, JP Buck had this new tape in his possession. By Tuesday afternoon, he was calling. *"Great job, Sean, very nice. I'll let you know how it goes. Very funny stuff."* OK—that hurdle was behind me. Now I could wait for the *real call*. The one I *really* wanted. The one that, unfortunately, *never came.*

It wasn't just me that was waiting. Every comic who had auditioned was feeling the same anxiety because Star Search was delaying their decision process until the very last minute. It wasn't until the last week of the year when the first comics were notified that they would be flying to Los Angeles to compete the very next week. Everyone knew exactly when the word came down because we were all glued to the stand-up message boards, just waiting to see who would go. We were like dogs in an over-crowded shelter, *pick me, pick me, hey, over here!*

Even though I wasn't selected for Star Search, the audition process gave me the confidence I needed. I had something good. I wouldn't have made it that far if I didn't possess the ability to shine. I did and this confirmed, reinforcing my confidence in my abilities and dreams. I wasn't giving up anytime soon and nobody wanted me to, really. I had support from family, friends, comedy clubs, and fellow comics. And just when this new level of confidence was starting to overflow, despite my long drawn-out Star Search rejection, I found a seemingly impossible opportunity with well-established comedian, Ralphie May.

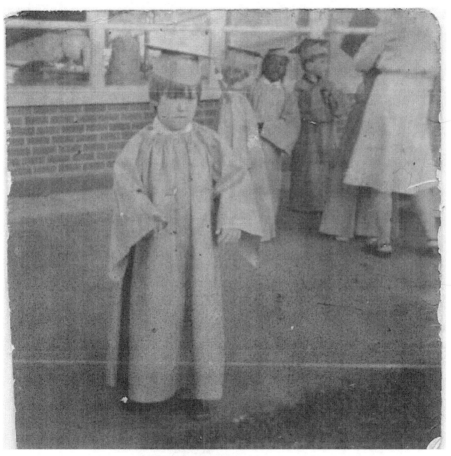

Four years old and graduating from the Head Start Program.
I was upset about something!

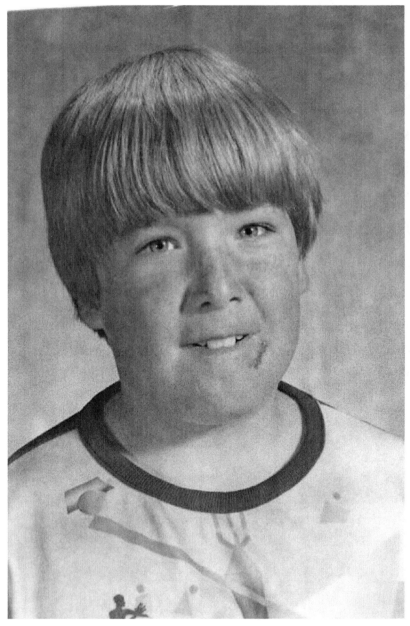

Seven or eight years old. "Husky" and growing.

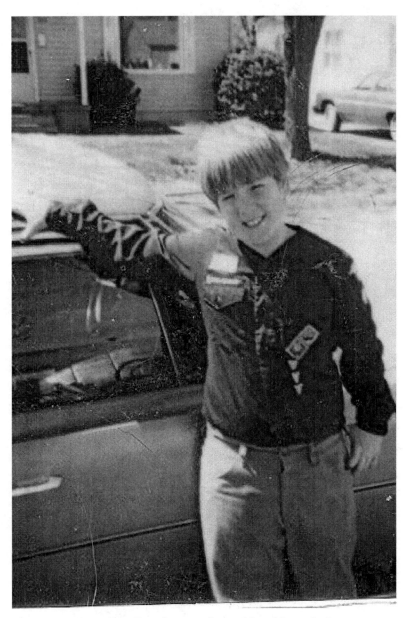

One of the few pictures of me with a shirt tucked.

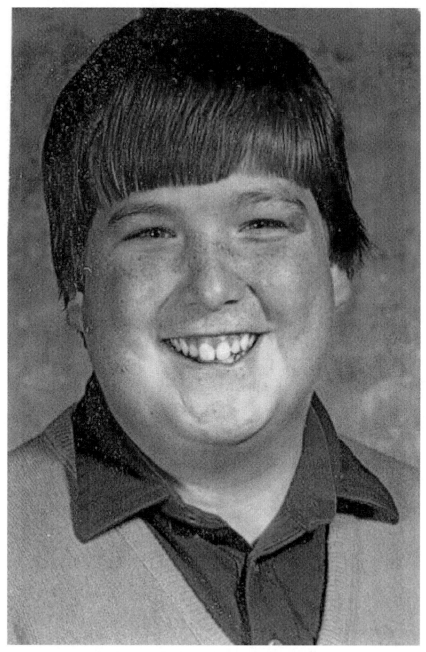

Twelve or thirteen here. My weight was quickly getting out of control.

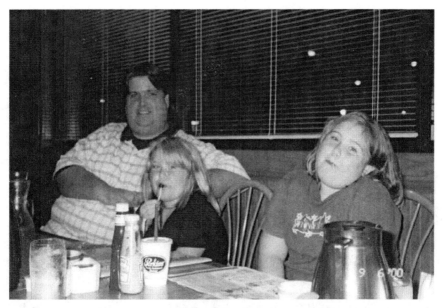

With my daughters!

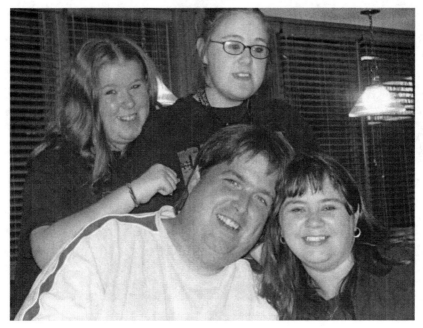

Our young family.

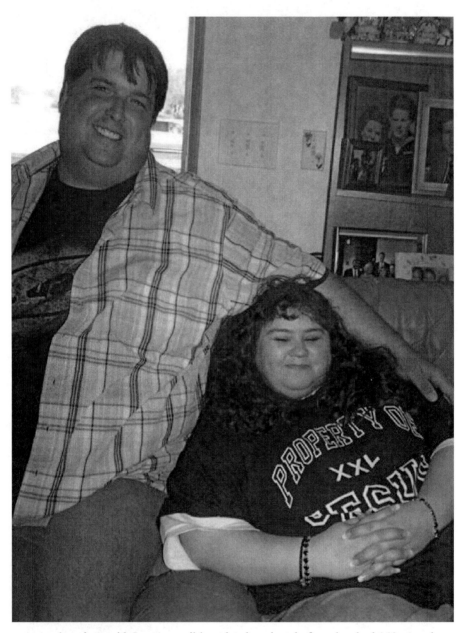

At my heaviest, with Irene, possibly at her heaviest, before she shed 140 pounds.

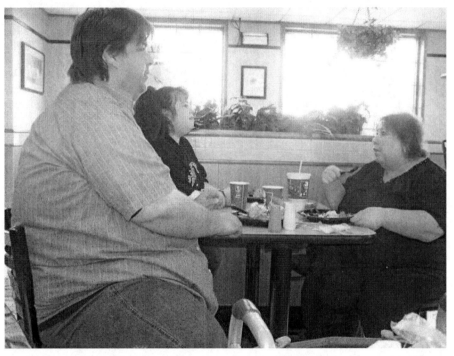

Very dramatic profile picture. Eating another fast food meal with mom and Irene.

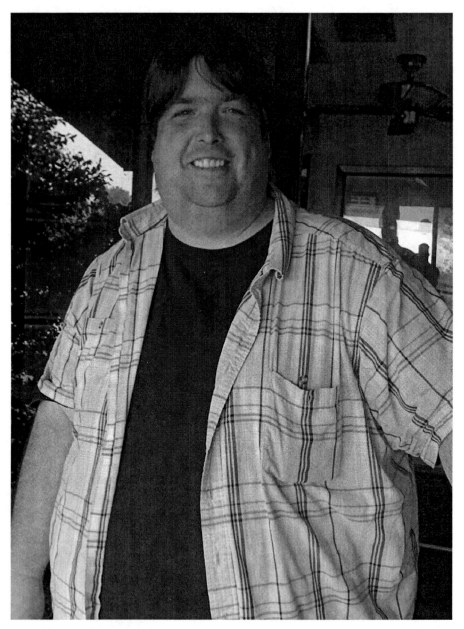

My broadcasting colleague Ryan Diamond snapped this 500 pound plus "before" picture with his phone. One of the biggest before pictures I have.

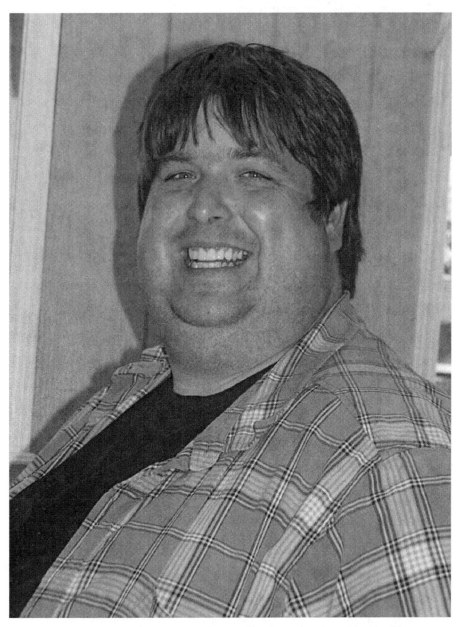

This shot was snapped by Aunt Kelli. It really shows just how big I had become.

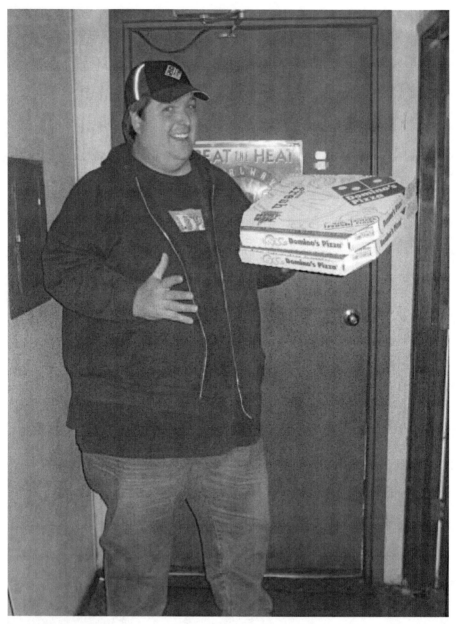

This was a KLOR radio public service campaign called, "Sean's Second Job For Toys." I delivered pizzas to raise money and buy gifts for kids in the domestic violence shelter.

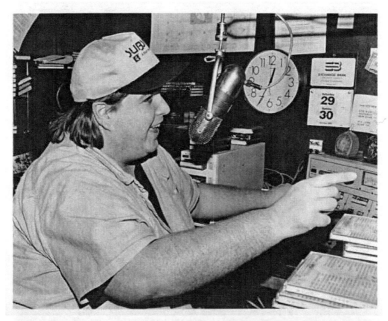

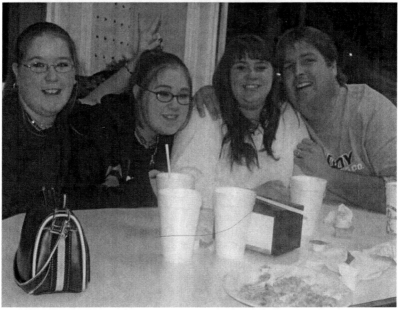

Top: In the studio of Star Country 1020 and Star 105.1 KASR Radio.
Photo credit: Jim Dunn Bottom: Posing for another restaurant family picture!

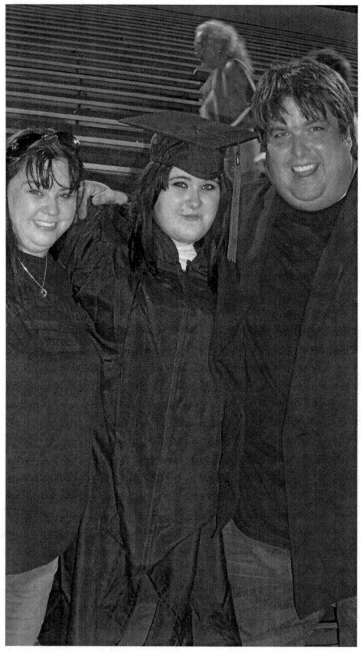

At Amber's high school graduation

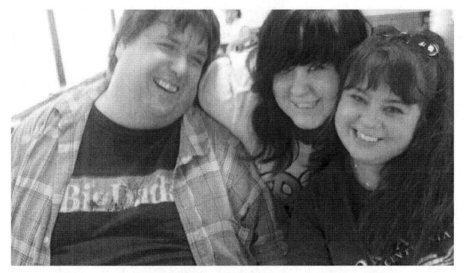

Me, Courtney, and Irene

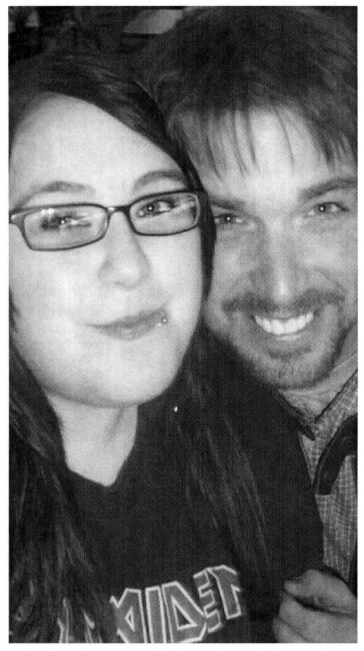

After Transformation with Amber

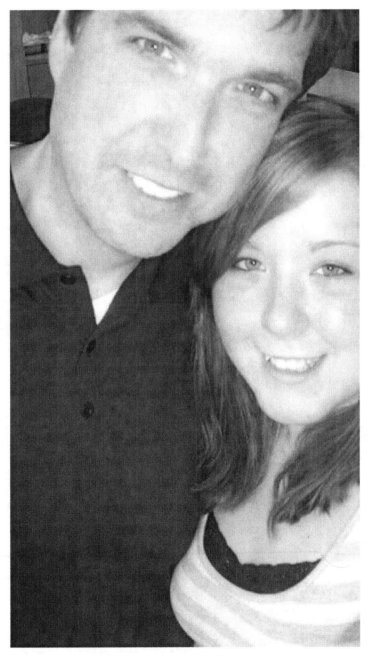

After Transformation with Courtney

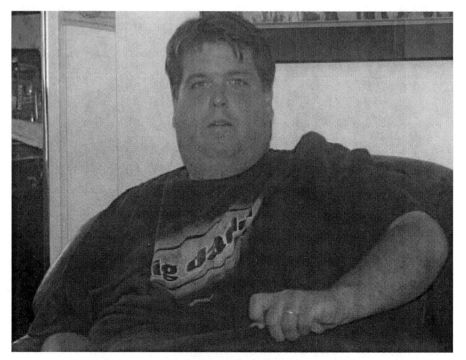

Big before picture—strange look.

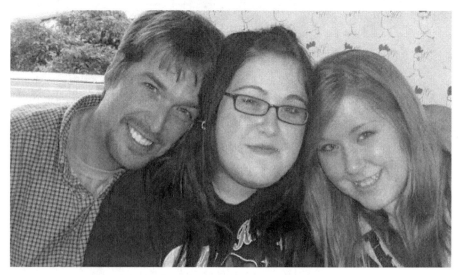

With my daughters after losing 275 pounds.

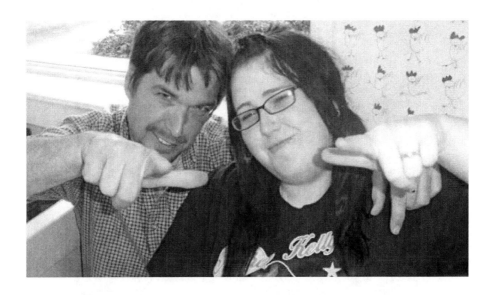

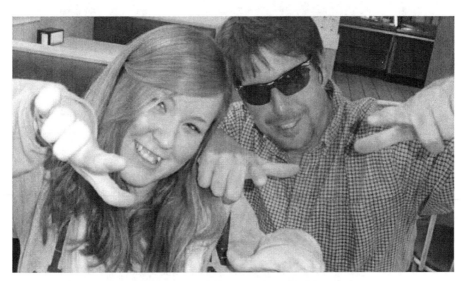

Sometimes, being silly is our favorite thing to do.
Two pictures, with our gangster gun pose on!

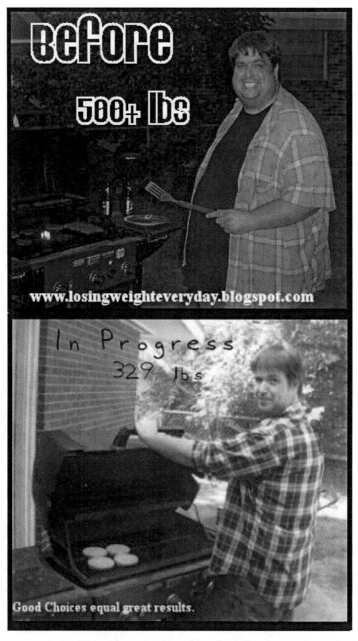

The dramatic "Grill-before and during" comparison photo. It was the first
comparison photo I shared on the blog.

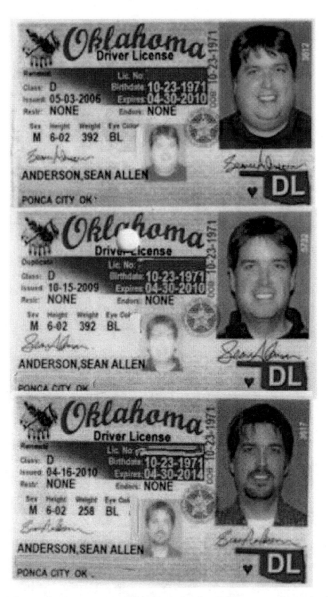

I never told the truth about my weight when getting a license--except in the bottom photo. The bottom of the three contains my actual weight at that moment. It was the first time I had ever been honest about my weight on an ID.

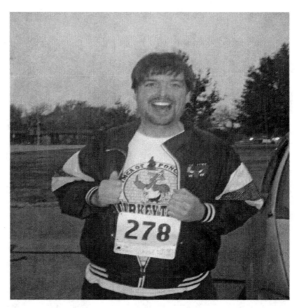

The YMCA Turkey Trot 10K, I did it!

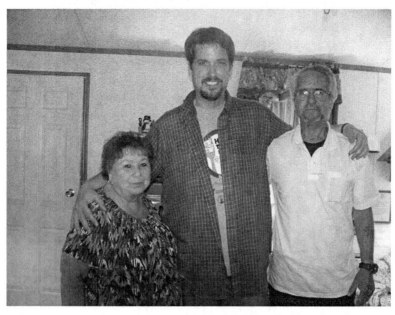

The first time ever to have both parents in the same room. I'll never forget that night. It was very strange.

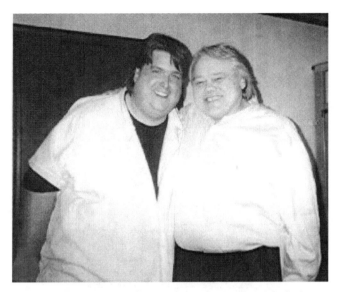

With fellow comedian Louie Anderson (no relation)

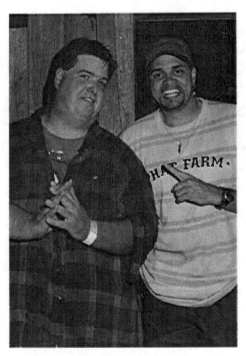

After opening for Sinbad at the thunderstorm plagued Orange Peel 1999.

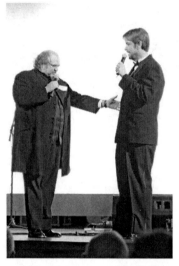

On the stage of the historic Poncan Theatre with Dave May.

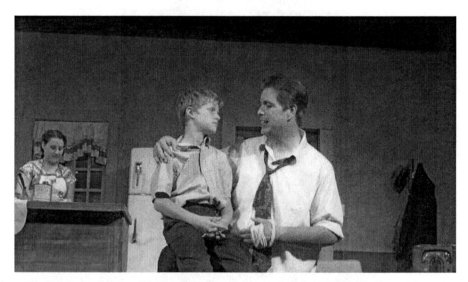

Realizing the dream of having a lead role in a stage play. With "Call Me Henry"
cast members Isaac Cervantes and Lauren Donahue.

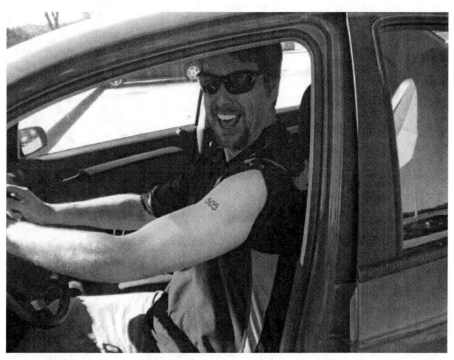

In my little red rental car, showing off the "505" tattoo to my friends Stephen Vinson and Tammy Ortagus while visiting in Alabama.

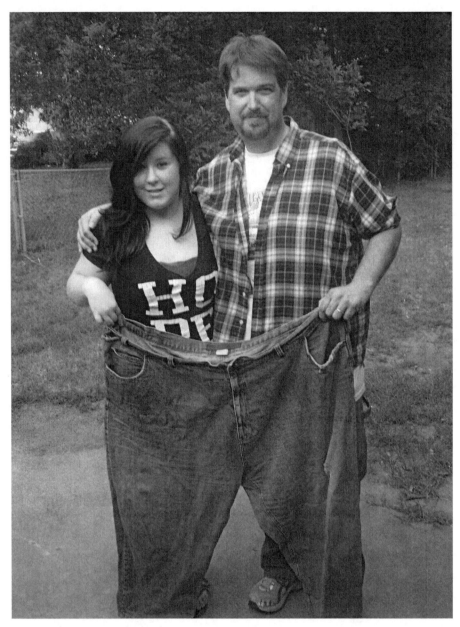

Along the way--nearly 200 pounds lost here--holding up the size 64's with Courtney--I think we could both fit inside these now!

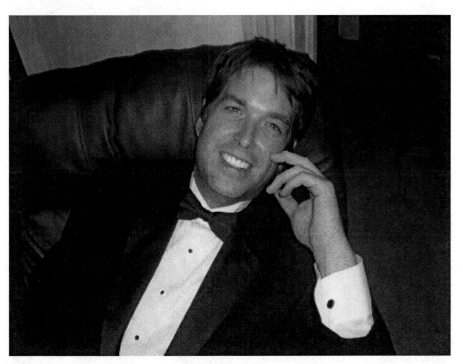

I never wore a tuxedo before I lost the weight, not even at my wedding. Now, I wear one as much as possible, thanks to the wonderful fitters at Spray's Jewelry and Tuxedos in downtown Ponca City, Oklahoma.

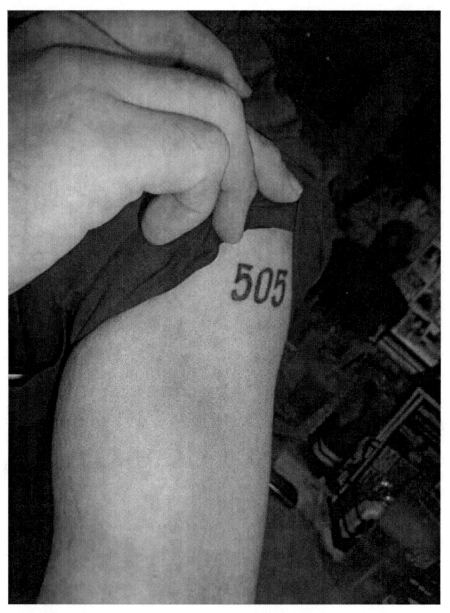

The tattoo artist who did this was over 460 pounds at the time. Not anymore, The very talented tattoo artist, Mike Springer has lost a couple hundred pounds too! And yes, he tells me he plans on getting a similar tattoo! It's a very simple tattoo, but a powerful reminder, everyday of my life.

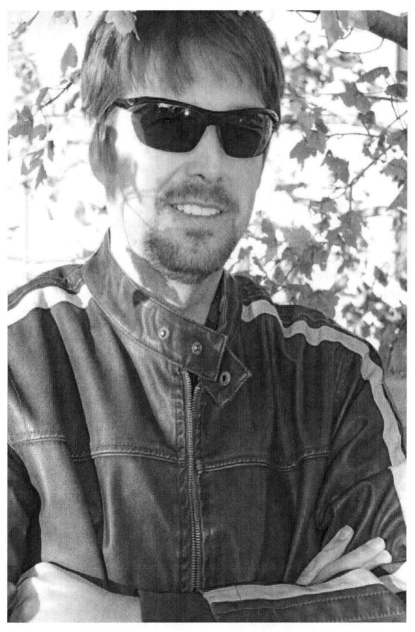

At my heaviest, I never liked the way sunglasses fit my giant face. Now, I love to wear them. One of the simple joys along the way!

Chapter Nineteen

Chasing the Dream

I knew of Ralphie. I had watched Ralphie on TV numerous times. I was in awe of Ralphie because like me, Ralphie was morbidly obese. He was doing it, succeeding despite his size in a town where good looks seemed to be a requirement. But in the world of stand-up, talent and personality trumped looks every time. Ralphie had it all, he was sharply tuned with an over-the-top attitude that spoke the truth. He wasn't pretending to be anything he wasn't or didn't like to be. He was in your face real, and his genuine realness and absolute fearless delivery of the truth, is why he was so successful. Of course, I say all of that in hindsight. I was convinced that I could be just as successful someday, if only I could get to where the industry lived and breathed: Hollywood. Oh, yeah, the opportunity with Ralphie, you see . . .

Ralphie and his girlfriend Lahna had mentioned on the stand-up message boards that they had an extra room available in their apartment for any comic that was ready to take the plunge in Los Angeles. I immediately started trying to figure out how that comic could be me. It was far-fetched, really. I was back with Irene and the girls and things were finally settling down from our separation. Besides, even if Irene and the girls gave me their blessing to pursue my dream in LA, there was no way we could afford to maintain two households. I needed a plan. I wasn't just going to let this pass by without trying to launch some kind of plan. The Star Search situation had given me a confidence level that needed to be in Los Angeles.

I immediately approached a friend and huge supporter A'kos Kovach. Ak owned a mortgage company in Stillwater. He first came to know me by listening to my radio show on a regular basis, and eventually he contributed characters to the show, like the weatherman-wrestler from the NWWS or the National Wrestling Weather Service, a character that delivered the radio weather like a wrestler trash talking before a big match. The funniest thing was when he would challenge our real meteorologist, Channel 4's David Payne, to a cage fight. This was the kind of radio that got me nominated for personality of the year. Ak was a big reason for that success. And Ak was absolutely one of my friends and one of my biggest fans.

Ak had hired me to do stand-up on several occasions, mainly at his annual company Christmas party. He's a big laugher and enjoys humor on a therapeutic level. He told me that laughter had been proven to add years to people's lives, so in doing what I was doing, I was helping people live longer. Ak knew all about my Star Search experience and when I told him about the opportunity with Ralphie in Los Angeles, he agreed that it could possibly be something huge.

Ak immediately realized that I was asking for his financial support of this dream and he told me to put together a business proposal. I did, treating it strictly like an investment. Nothing too elaborate, just enough to keep me in a bedroom while I worked my way into the business of Los Angeles stand-up. With Irene and the girls giving me their blessing and with Ak's investment in me, I was on my way. I secured the room with Ralphie and to give myself extra money, I managed to book gigs in Amarillo, Albuquerque and Santa Fe for the trip out West. I gave Team Radio short notice to end my part-time commitment and they wished me well. It was happening. I was on my way. This was exciting!

My stop in Amarillo was familiar ground. I had performed at the Amarillo Comedy Club more than a half a dozen times. It was a nice confidence booster at the beginning of this journey. I just couldn't believe that I was on my way. After a great week at Laffs Comedy

Club in Albuquerque, I enjoyed back-to-back bookings at New Mexico casinos. The second casino was the big one just South of Albuquerque and they put me up at the beautiful Wyndham Hotel. After an amazing show, I opened the curtains in my fifteenth-story room overlooking the lights of the city and I just laid on the bed taking it all in. The only thing that could have made the moment better? Ice cream!

This place had a concierge, so I just knew I could get some ice cream, somehow, someway. Well, the concierge wasn't on duty, but the front desk guy gave me the bad news. The restaurant was closed. If I really wanted ice cream, I would need to drive somewhere. The disappointment in my voice must have hit this guy right in the heart. Maybe he was an ice cream addict, too, I don't know, but what he did next was certainly above and beyond the call of duty. He told me he would see what he could do and within minutes he was at my door with a quart of Haagen-Dazs and a real silver spoon. Not a pint, but a quart. Not aluminum, but big heavy silver. He told me that he had swiped it from the closed restaurant kitchen. What a guy, putting his job on the line in order to feed my addiction. I graciously tipped him a whole two dollars. *What? That wasn't enough for ten bucks worth of stolen super premium ice cream served with a silver spoon in my hotel room at one AM?* OK, you're right, it wasn't enough. But I didn't have change, and isn't it impolite to ask for change while tipping? I was new at this stuff. I had never stayed at a hotel that would have given me a donut at one AM, let alone a quart of Haagen-Dazs. If I ever see that guy again, I'll slip him a five-spot.

How many calories are in a quart of super premium vanilla Haagen-Dazs? I don't know. And I didn't care to look. I didn't need the buzz-kill, I was high on vanilla bean, baby. I flipped through the channels, occasionally glanced out at my wonderful view of Albuquerque, and consumed every last creamy drop of that amazing ice cream. I was on my way to the good life, and it all started appropriately with a quart of Haagen-Dazs and a silver spoon.

My food addiction and compulsive eating didn't waste any time realizing the freedom that the road and a lonely hotel room provided. Our little secret was safe. That entire large pizza in Amarillo? Nobody had to know. The family size bag of Nacho Cheese Doritos that slowly disappeared along the way? *Shhhh!* The ten dollars worth of Taco Cabana at two AM? *I never thought it would be mentioned in a book.* And that quart of Haagen-Dazs that only me and a soon-to-be-unemployed hotel worker knew about were all sure signs that my mind was the furthest it had ever been from caring about my weight.

What's really puzzling to any reasonable person is how I knew that losing weight would greatly benefit my swollen right leg, but still, I carelessly pressed on. Sure, it's just a part of the prison of obesity. I knew life would be better on the "outside," but as long as the symptoms were manageable, I could go on ignoring the problem and just surviving. That course was much easier than dealing with the issues of food addiction and compulsive eating.

My right leg wasn't going to be manageable very long. The swelling was a constant reminder of my horrible condition. The sores would start developing again, and this time, Irene wouldn't be there to nurse me back to health. Instead, I had a bottle of Vicodin prescribed to me by a dentist, all ready to go, in case the sores and resulting pain started. And it was just a matter of time, because at over 500 pounds, I couldn't physically wrap my own leg with the compression bandages. Without the wrapping or constant elevation, the pressure and swelling on my right leg was too much. Irene wrapped me every day to keep the swelling under control and the sores away. Even when we were separated, I would occasionally show up with bandages in hand and she would wrap me, even if her new boyfriend was in the next room. She cared too much to not help, even if her new man thought we were crazy. And now, we were back together, but I was going to be fourteen hundred miles away. I really didn't think this through too well.

If this move was a bad idea or not, it didn't matter, it was happening. There was no turning back. I finished my gigs in New

Mexico and hit I-40 for the West Coast. I made plans to audition for NBC's Last Comic Standing just a few days into this adventure. The first thing I did when I rolled into town was eat at a Kentucky Fried Chicken. *Can you believe that?* I drive clear across the country and the first thing I do is visit KFC. The second thing I did was look for my exit off of I-10. Crenshaw, *Crenshaw Boulevard.* Hmmm, *where had I heard that street name before?* Oh, my, in gangster rap songs about gang warfare! I was a little nervous because seriously, I was coming from a place voted to be one of the safest cities in America and moving straight into South Central LA. I remember Ralphie joking about living in the hood, but come on, *wasn't that just a joke?* I should have remembered, Ralphie didn't do anything that wasn't real, if he said he lived in the hood, that's where I was headed.

The apartment was an upstairs apartment in a two-story house-like dwelling with a staircase in the front and back. It was on fifth, just off of Adams, and down the street from Crenshaw. The neighborhood really wasn't that bad. It wasn't what I imagined at all. Maybe it's the palm trees that made it look nice or the fact that every lawn looked perfectly manicured. I was fully expecting helicopters and gunshots, instead it was quiet, nice, and felt relatively safe. It was getting late and I was the only one home because Ralphie and Lahna were performing in Hawaii. But they left me turn-by-turn directions to some major points of interest that they knew I would want to visit right away.

The next day I headed straight for the Hollywood Improv on Melrose. I needed to drop off an audition video for Stu, the talent guy. I pulled up and just sat there in my car across the street, staring at the sign and the building and pinching myself. This was the place where I had dreamed of performing. This was the World Famous Hollywood Improv. I watched A&E's *An Evening at the Improv* when I was a kid and this was the place! I must have been fixed on the building for fifteen minutes before I decided to go inside.

I was in awe of everything, everywhere. A trip over to Sunset and the Comedy Store had me all excited. I had heard of the stories about this place, legendary stories! And there it was, right in front of my eyes. I was determined to make a mark in this town and the first thing was an audition at NBC in Burbank for a new show called Last Comic Standing.

When Ralphie returned from Hawaii, I excitedly told him all about my plans to audition for the show. He was very supportive, but quickly reminded me that one of his best friends was Jay Mohr, the host and creator of the show. Ralphie had a special invitation audition along with several other prominent comics in town. He was pretty sure that he was getting on the show and the chances of the producers picking two "big" comics was next to zero. I appreciated Ralphie's straightforward advice and decided that the experience would be worth it regardless.

Ralphie was right and so was I. It was worth the experience. I grew up watching the Tonight Show with Johnny Carson, so imagine my giddiness when I found out that the auditions were taking place on the old sound stage for the Tonight Show. I watched so many comics make their national television debut on that stage and I was going to audition in the same room. Wow. My excitement turned to disoriented confusion when it was my turn to perform.

I was told to walk through the giant doors and keep walking toward the light, climb the stairs up to a platform stage and be ready. The sound stage was huge and empty. It looked nothing like I remember, and of course it wouldn't, the set was long gone. But this was the legendary space and that was good enough to thrill me. My short set was cut short with a simple, "thank you." Wow, this wasn't anything like my Star Search experience. I was one and done, *just happy to be there.*

When Stu with the Improv called and invited me to perform on the New Faces show, I didn't realize just how exclusive it was. He told me he liked my tape and he would see how I did with the New Faces. I later ran across comics that had been trying to get on the New Faces show forever, so I was really honored and pumped that things were happening so quickly. I was in awe of performing in front of that same brick wall I had seen on TV years ago, when I would stay up late with Mom, laughing until way past my bedtime.

After two performances at the Improv's New Faces show, Stu approached me and said those magical words: *"You can start calling in for regular spots as one of the host MC comedians."* I felt like a ball player who just got called up to the majors. I was going to be a paid regular at the Hollywood Improv and I had been in town less than a month at that point. This was a big deal to me.

I imagine a rookie ball player sitting on the bench next to people like Derek Jeter and Alex Rodriguez feels much like I did at my first professional Improv show. I was hosting the show, doing my set first and then introducing every single comic after. Big names, all in the same live show: Dave Chappelle, Damon Wayans, George Wallace, Harland Williams, Zach Galifianakis, Costaki Economopoulos, and me. *Me!! It was surreal.* I was so stressed out trying to remember how to pronounce Galifianakis and Economopoulos. George Wallace was the nicest and most approachable of them all. He actually spent about twenty minutes outside on the sidewalk asking me questions about Oklahoma and my experiences in stand-up.

My experiences in stand-up mostly included me making fun of myself. But I wouldn't focus on that at all. When asked, I would talk about the wonderful connection with the audience, the natural high of making an audience erupt in laughter, and how blessed I was to be pursuing something with such passion. And I was passionate about those things, it just came at a high price. I was my own bully at this point. I was in Hollywood and representing myself as this big, fun, lovable fat guy, who was completely at peace with his size and role as such. *Wasn't this what I wanted?* If I was constantly searching for acceptance of my 500-pound self, I was finding it, but how can one feel real love and acceptance from others without honestly loving and accepting himself first?

I thought that I was being genuine, I really did. However, over the years and countless shows, my true feelings about my material and self would be reflected in audience members who would occasionally approach me after a show. They were most usually obese themselves and they were deeply disturbed by some of my material. Maybe it was a certain look I gave, something wasn't right, and they could tell. My acceptance of this self-deprecating material wasn't believable to them. They could see the pain through the laughter and they just wanted to let me know how it made them feel.

I would smile and tell them that it was alright, *it's just comedy!* Then I would walk away knowing that they knew *the real me.* I really felt the same way they did, disturbed, but I was glad that only one or two percent of the audience could sense this underlying truth. Because the show must go on and I had a show to do!

I must be a decent actor because I was convincing. I even convinced myself that I was fine with it all, until opportunity made me face my true feelings about the character I portrayed, much like those affected audience members, except this time I couldn't just walk away, I had to admit that it wasn't cool to me. There was a limit and I was about to discover it.

Chapter Twenty

Living the Dream

Valentine's Day in 2003 found me alone at the apartment. I was thinking about Irene and the girls and how I wasn't there with them on this special day. I was also thinking about my little brother Shane who would have been twenty-six on this day. My somber mood was suddenly interrupted with a phone call from Ralphie, telling me that I needed to call the Kimmel Show and speak with a producer. Ralphie had put in a good word for me and suddenly, a national TV show was interested in taking my call. I immediately perked up, cleared my throat, and practiced saying, *"This is Sean Anderson, Ralphie May told me to call."* My excitement quickly turned sour while talking with the producer from the Kimmel Show.

As a special comedic opening segment to their Valentine's show, they wanted to have a fat guy dressed up like Cupid, prancing up the sidewalk along Hollywood Boulevard, just outside the El Capitan theater studios. If I wanted the job, it was mine. I would be required to wear a giant diaper, wings, a halo, and nothing else. I immediately said I wasn't available. I didn't want to know what I would be paid because it didn't matter, and it wasn't an option. I couldn't do this, *what about my right leg?* The swelling and painful sores were once again out of control and the secret about them was always safely hidden under the pants leg of my jeans. Accepting this opportunity wasn't an option simply because of that fact.

But really, there was this deeper issue I was starting to recognize. I wasn't comfortable being the fat guy-clown. My food addiction

146

behaviors kept me at 500 pounds and I adapted and survived. I pretended to be fine with my weight in front of others, but now I was realizing something very scary. I couldn't stand myself but felt powerless to change. The stress and emotions that these feelings created made me want to eat even more because everything would be great while I was eating. I needed to eat more and more, so everything would be great more and more of the time.

Facing who I really was and how I really felt was too scary and pressure-filled. A bunch of people believed in me. My family, my friends, my fellow comics, and the dear friend in Ak, who was generously keeping me afloat financially while I found my place in the city of lights. I was finding myself faster than I was finding my place, but what that meant to fully embrace, just wasn't an option in my mind. I had to press on. I had to find as much stage time as possible so I could get better *and get discovered.* Saying no to a national TV show on a major network probably wasn't a step in that direction, but it was a necessary step in the direction of being honest with myself. And that was something far more important.

"Who got you, Kimmel? That's right, man, you haven't been in town two months and you're getting on TV, you're welcome." Ralphie was excited and happy to help me as he quickly reminded me how unusual it was and how fortunate the situation. *"Ralphie, I told them I couldn't do it."* *"What's wrong with you? Are you crazy?"* *"No, I just, well, the whole diaper thing, I would have been too embarrassed."* I honestly can't remember Ralphie's response to this, but it's safe to say it was puzzled disbelief mixed with a little disgust. I hadn't shown Ralphie my messed up right leg, nobody in the world, except Irene and Dr. Hill had laid eyes on it in this condition. Not even my mom and daughters, that's how protective I was about this increasing problem. If I had shown Ralphie, he probably would have understood. He probably would have told me to go home and get well. Home, *as in Stillwater.*

147

My goal was to make "home" in California. I needed to find a way to get Irene and the girls with me. I needed something steady, a job, and lucky for me, Westwood One Radio Networks was hiring. I was very confident in my broadcasting talent and abilities. I sent a tape to the program director of the 24/7 Oldies format satellite service, and it didn't take long for him to call me in for an interview. *This could be HUGE,* I thought. Never mind that I didn't have any major market experience, just give me a chance and I'll wow you. That's the thought that fueled my confidence.

The drive to Valencia was exciting. I was confident and daydreaming about possibly making Valencia a home for my family. If I could land this high-paying part-time job, it would enable me to make ends meet with everything else, and I could send for the girls. I would still have time to do stand-up and pursue my career, and everything would be perfect. I arrived in Valencia early, so I had lunch at a Burger King, just down the road from Magic Mountain. I scarfed down several hundred calories in an attempt to calm my nerves. My weight was the least of my concerns at that moment. I was going into that interview with an almost delusional confidence and a full stomach. Nothing could shake my zone. Well, except maybe the most embarrassing chair breaking incident of my entire life.

Rick Santos was one of the program directors at Westwood One. This guy was the gatekeeper. If I impressed him, then I would land the best job of my broadcasting career. He greeted me in the lobby and was all smiles. We talked as he took me on an amazing tour of their headquarters. The studios were lining the halls, each fascinating me. I was wide-eyed excited. I was doing my best to contain myself and maintain an air of professionalism, not wanting to seem too eager. And Rick seemed to like me, not even remotely concerned or shocked by my 500-pound self. He was an old radio pro, surely he had worked with people of similar size. In radio, you're either naturally thin, or overweight. There's hardly ever any in between. It's a sedentary job, after all. A bunch of sitting. Good chairs are an important thing in a broadcasting facility.

After the tour, Rick invited me into his office for the interview. I walked in and immediately realized that this was going to be a challenge. The two chairs in front of his desk had arms. I had spent my entire life avoiding chairs with narrow arms and, now, I had to pick one that I knew I wouldn't fit into. I was just hoping to squeeze myself into the seat and hold my breath long enough to get through the interview. I paused for a moment and then he asked me to have a seat. I sat down as lightly as I could, but nothing was going to make my 500 pounds any less taxing on this particle board and hot glued chair. *This is Westwood One Radio Networks, shouldn't the chairs be solid wood?* The chair didn't even give me a second. As soon as I squeezed in between the narrow arms, it immediately *exploded underneath.* There was no fixing this chair. It was destroyed, much like my chances of landing this dream job. This wasn't my first chair breaking incident, but it was absolutely the most unfortunate and embarrassing chair failure of my life.

Rick was such a nice guy. He immediately told me not to worry about it and offered the other chair. The other chair, *the one identical to the pile of particle board and cushion on the floor.* This could have been worse. The second chair was obviously the least used because somehow it survived my weight. Of course, I sat on the edge, putting all of my weight on my feet. I was miserable, embarrassed, and completely distracted from my focus. I don't even remember the interview because I was so overwhelmed with horror over the chair breaking. Rick seemed to be fine with the experience, but still, he never called me back. I wonder how many times he's re-told that story. Once again, my obesity was trying to get my attention, but if my bad leg couldn't spark something, then all this experience would do is give me more weight-related material on the stand-up stages of LA.

My leg situation was a convenient excuse for me to not deal with the real issue of me getting tired of making my size the punch line. I really had enough at this point. I found myself in a situation where my addiction and compulsive eating were out of control, my emotions were in shambles, and I felt like I had no choice but to continue the charade. But I wanted to continue the funny on my own terms and not on the terms of the industry, of which I so badly craved acceptance. I was in an all-around messed up mental dynamic. And now, I wasn't sure if Ralphie would be as willing to help me, considering how I just blew off the Kimmel people. And I was pretty sure the Kimmel show wouldn't be calling or taking my calls again anytime soon.

While I started discovering my deepest feelings about everything, I started discovering new and tasty sources to feed my food addiction. Popeye's Chicken and Biscuits, In-N-Out Burger, Jack in the Box, and Del Taco were places we didn't have back home and they were quickly becoming some of my favorite escapes. I'd rush in, buy as much as I wanted, then swiftly head back to the apartment and feast. Nothing like a Double Double, fries, and a shake, or a big bag of Del Taco—or both—to make me feel like everything was right and good.

Everything was far from being right and good, and if the pain in my right leg wasn't reminding me, then Pimp, Ralphie and Lahna's dog would. Pimp knew something wasn't right with my leg because his keen sense of smell drew him to it every time. I was so worried that people would notice the attention and fascination Pimp seemed to have with my pants leg. Yeah, Pimp knew what was going on. It's hard to fool a dog. It's much easier to fool others *and myself.*

Chapter Twenty-One

Killing the Dream

W hen homesickness and the pain and swelling became too much to handle, I found a way and a reason to drive back home and see my family. I needed to see Dr. Hill for my usual healing prescriptions of Augmenten XR and Silvadeen cream, and then have Irene work her magic at nursing me back to health. We counted over a dozen open sores, a few as big as an inch across and a quarter inch deep. It was bad. But this medicine and Irene were good. With me on my back, leg elevated, medicine in me and the sores being treated—I was miraculously healed during this four-day pit stop. *Four days!* Of course, it was a temporary fix because I was headed right back into the race, far away from the daily wrapping and attention I needed to keep it in check. And even further away from any spark of weight loss interest that would ultimately help the condition.

I had booked a weekend of performances in Amarillo for the return trip and I hit that Texas stage with a renewed confidence and overall attitude. I wasn't in Amarillo long when my phone rang with an unfamiliar 323 area code number. It was a Jimmy Kimmel Live producer. I couldn't believe that he was still interested in working with me after my Valentine's Day decline, but there I was, face to face with another request, and this time it had me questioning myself. *Could I be paid enough to swallow my pride and insecurities?*

The producer described the premise of this latest elaborate skit. It would be called *"The Fatchelor."* The show wanted a morbidly obese man to be surrounded by bikini-clad women, all fawning over and competing for his attention. Instead of roses, the Fatchelor would hand out donuts or something along those lines. Again, the punch line would be my size, but this time it wouldn't be a one shot non-speaking cold open. Not at all. This time it would be a fully produced series of skits, twelve to eighteen appearances over the course of a month, with "couch time" alongside Jimmy after each airing. We're talking thousands of dollars. And considering my financial situation at the time, there's no way I could possibly turn it down. Saying yes to this meant possibly hurting my already fragile marriage, simply because of the premise, even though I would be acting, and it also meant I would have to share my limitations and concerns with the director and producers, and hope they would understand and accommodate.

I immediately agreed to do it, deciding to work out the potential conflicts later. I told the gentleman on the phone that I would be back in town on Monday and ready to go. He then informed me that this wouldn't wait till then, and I needed to be at the studio within two hours. They wanted the first installment on the air that night. And since I didn't have access to a personal leer jet, it was impossible. Knowing what was on the line, financially, I tried to reason with the producer. I told him that I was working on the road, but I would be back Monday with a clear schedule of LA-area-only gigs. If the show could wait for me, I promised to make it worth the delay. The show wasn't waiting. I was in Amarillo making a couple hundred bucks when I should have been in LA making thousands. Jimmy Kimmel's impatience might have cost me, but it might have saved me in other ways. Still, I had the displeasure of obsessing over this missed opportunity the rest of the weekend. And after watching the show and seeing who they used, I couldn't help but think, *that was supposed to be me.*

It didn't take long to realize that aside from my occasional paid gigs, I needed a real job. Westwood One wasn't calling and the occasional Improv booking was laughable money because it was a "showcase" club, I should have been *paying them* to perform on that stage. Doug James was booking me from Bakersfield to Orange County and everywhere in between, but still, I was opening, not headlining. In order to survive, I had to work *somewhere*. And the fantasy that the Kimmel Show would swoop in to save me with another opportunity like the one I had just missed, was just that, fantasy, *wishful thinking*. Through my connections in stand-up, I discovered a part-time job in telephone sales with the state theater of California, The Pasadena Playhouse. It was a job that was performer friendly, allowing flexibility when and if opportunity struck. And to my surprise, an opportunity with the Kimmel Show came again in late June.

I don't even remember asking what they wanted, I just said yes and *"when should I arrive?"* That was a very risky thing to do considering the previous requests. The one thing I was certain of was my size would be the punch line, whatever they wanted me to do. I was told to be there as soon as possible and before I could end the call, I was on my way to Hollywood Boulevard. I couldn't believe they were giving me a third chance. *Was Hollywood really that short of morbidly obese actors or comedians?* I arrived and was briefed on the premise and plan.

Airports had just introduced the new full-body scanners that would allow airport security to *see* your undergarments. This comedy bit would include me and a couple of former "juggies" from Kimmel's "The Man Show," posing as audience members entering the studio through a full-body scanner. The women would walk into the scanner, revealing their panties and bras on the display screen. Then, I would follow, and you would see that I was also wearing women's undergarments. Comedy gold, my friend, comedy gold. *Oh, boy.*

The director pulled me aside and told me that I would need to go upstairs with a photographer for a picture of me wearing a giant bra and panties. When I immediately balked, he assured me that the photo would be turned into a negative and barely recognizable as me, except for the outline of the out-stretched undergarments. This was a breaking point for me. *I refused.*

153

"If that is what you need from me to be a part of this skit, I'll walk right now." I wasn't being easy to work with and that was something so out of character. The director wasn't happy, but he didn't fire me. Instead, he left to talk it over with Jimmy, and when he returned I was sure that Jimmy would have ordered me off the set, but he didn't. I was still in the skit and they would use an overweight production assistant as a stand-in for the fake scan picture. Imagine that, I *needed* a stand-in to accommodate my insecurities and modesty. The bit was taking forever to produce and eventually we were informed that it would be ready for air the next night. In the meantime, I was invited to hang around the greenroom and take in the experience of the show. I was in awe of everything.

The greenroom was divided into two rooms, one for games, and the other for food and drinks. Private dressing rooms, reserved for the guest stars, were just around the corner and upstairs. The video games were all set to "free play." I didn't even know that setting existed on a Galaga machine. *Wow!* The catering was all high-end stuff you would find in the fanciest of restaurants. I was very picky, sticking with anything that looked deep fried, and avoiding the healthy-looking stuff. The bar was open and free. Whatever you wanted, pick your poison, it was on the house.

Ralphie had casually warned me about acting star-struck, it just wasn't cool. After all, I was a professional, *right?* Considering that one of my favorite movies of all time is *Back to the Future,* imagine how crazy excited I was to see Crispen Glover casually chatting with someone just a few feet away. And, oh, my goodness, that's Carson Daly over there! *Be cool, be cool. You're one of them, kind of, not really, but keep it under control regardless.* I was invited back to hang out the next night, too, but had to decline because I was booked for a show more than two hours away at a club in an Eastern California desert town. If the timing was right, I could do that stand-up gig, then find a TV to watch my national TV debut.

I've always found clarity in my thoughts while driving. Some of my best material was written in my head while driving. It was quiet time within, giving me introspective insight into my most bare and honest feelings. That drive through the Mojave Desert made me think about where I was, what I was doing, and where I was headed. I had promised Irene and the girls that it wouldn't be long before I could get myself in position to bring them out and we would live an ideal life in Glendale or some other town *that wasn't named Los Angeles.* The problem was, I could clearly see the truth. And the truth was, it might take much longer to reach that point, much longer than I expected, longer than Ak, who by now found himself fighting for his life and eventually winning the battle against colon cancer, had signed up for, and way longer than my family could wait without me.

I became a better man during that two-and-a-half-hour drive. I thought about what was really important in life. I thought about how I was raised without my father present in my life and the issues that it created inside me, issues I didn't want my girls to have. I thought about how uncomfortable I was playing the role of the big guy. I dreamed of losing weight someday, although at the time, the possibility of that happening seemed just as elusive as comedic stardom. I had to step out of my dream long enough to see what I was doing and try to understand the possible consequences of my choices. There was a really good chance it wasn't going to end well and I just couldn't afford to take that chance.

My mind was nearly made up by the time I hit the stage that night; I was going home soon. I had to get back to reality and my family. They needed me and I desperately needed them. It was a disconnected enthusiasm that engulfed me as everyone gathered around the bar that night to watch Jimmy Kimmel Live. *There I was, on TV!* All of my family and friends were back home watching, none of them ever imagining the decision I was about to announce.

I made two calls the next day, one to Irene and one to Mr. Bill Coleman, owner of Team Radio, a four-time employer of yours truly.

Irene cried tears of joy upon hearing my revelations and she told me that she was proud of me and she supported my decisions in whatever I wanted to do. Bill did not cry tears of joy. I think Bill was slightly confused and more than a little reserved and concerned about my inquiring of possible openings. I was a real wild card to Bill, he knew that I could be whatever he needed me to be, but would I be reliable enough for him to gamble a fifth round of employment?

Lucky for me, Bill and Jerry were displeased just enough with the current morning show personality on KLOR that taking another chance on me sounded like a decent idea. Bill told me to give him thirty days. He wanted to help the other guy get hired somewhere else (yes, Bill really is that nice of a boss. *Hey, I really want to fire you, but first, let me help you find another job. Where else, but Team Radio?*) and then it would be open for me, but this time, I better give him "at least one year" of committed service and it would require me to move my family to Ponca City. It all sounded really good to me.

It didn't sound as good to my close comedy buddy Cruz Carr. We had a pact. Whoever made it to California first, would help the other when they were ready to make the trip. At the same time I was preparing to make the trip home, he was ready to make the trip out West. This wasn't going to be good. He had just witnessed me in a comedy bit on Jimmy Kimmel Live, he knew I was a regular at the Hollywood Improv and I was getting booked all over the place. I had connections that were growing, connections that were prematurely promised to help him out someday, just as he would do for me if it were the other way around. In his eyes, I was on the brink of something big *at any moment.* But my perspective was a little clearer.

The confrontation at a truck stop in the middle of Arizona, or was it New Mexico? I can't remember. I do remember it was a very interesting meeting to say the least. He was hurt really, but refused to show that emotion. He was too macho for that, but I could tell. His anger spewed with obscenities at how crazy stupid I was for leaving. And I felt horrible because I was doing this to him, but I didn't have a choice. Cruz didn't have children or a wife and Cruz didn't fully understand my reluctance to be something that I had pretended to be for the duration of our friendship. It was confusing for him and very unfortunate. He thought I was absolutely insane, but I was actually thinking clearer than I had in a very long time. I would make some calls on his behalf, but this wasn't what we agreed on all of these years. I was leaving him high and dry and really, it signaled the end of our friendship as we knew it, for a very long time. We've since made peace with each other, but we rarely speak. Cruz is a successful private investigator and as far as I know, he still occasionally finds a stage to unleash his funny, often enraged brand of stand-up.

My friend and supporter A'kos Kovach was really in the position of being the most disappointed about this sudden change of heart and plans. Ak believed in me and never stopped believing in me. His gracious acceptance, amid slight confusion about my decision, was a peaceful way to end the arrangement we shared. It wasn't the outcome we were looking for, or thought I wanted, but it was definitely a lesson learned for both parties. I felt ashamed for letting down my friend, but Ak always has a wonderful way of putting things in perspective. When I expressed that someday I would be successful, he quickly jumped all over me, reminding me that I was successful in so many wonderful ways, the most important, being a father. Ak was incredibly insightful and philosophical, a quality that grew even more following his successful fight against colon cancer. He has an amazing wife, and he's an incredibly talented writer who is living, working, and writing in Arizona. I'll always call him a friend and I hope to someday sit, smile, and talk further about our experiences and where they have brought us.

Ralphie and Lahna were very good to me during my time in LA. They both ended up with stand-up material concerning my stay. Lahna wrote a song about the time I used her bar soap in the shower. She claimed it was disgusting because she washed her face with that soap, the same bar I undoubtedly used to wash my, uh, *you know*. My defense: Doesn't soap wash itself? The layer that was touching me has washed away by the time it would touch her pretty face. Anyway, it was a good argument, *I thought.*

And Ralphie, I've heard, but haven't confirmed, has a bit about the time I got into his pan of cooling brownies, only to discover they weren't your ordinary everyday brownies. I love brownies. *Doesn't everybody?* Especially warm, moist, fresh from-the-oven brownies, cut into small one inch squares. I thought enjoying three or four was reasonable, but apparently it was shocking and hilarious to everyone at the party. Ralphie never gave me the recipe and that's probably a good thing.

A friend of mine once asked if I was ever jealous of Ralphie's success. Before I knew him, yes. I would see him on TV and think to myself—*Look at him, he's morbidly obese like me. Hey, I can do that too and I can do it better!* After getting to know him during my short stay, I could clearly see the absurdity of my ridiculous thought process. Ralphie May *was and is* a star. He had honed his skills, paying dues for years and it had put him on an elite level in the comedy clubs that mattered in LA. I was honest enough to realize that Ralphie possessed a comic talent, *a brutal honesty* that I didn't.

Ralphie deserved every success coming his way and more, based on his hard work, exceptional talent, and willingness to generously help those around him. My meager success in Los Angeles was mainly based on being large and available. Had I been accepting of my size and role, completely honest and pure with my material, and a little more shameless, I could have gotten a lot of work. Ralphie was and is the real deal and I was still searching for my "real" self, and the difference between the two are galaxies apart, regardless of how similar we might have been in size.

Ralphie was extremely generous to this dreamer from Oklahoma. He opened doors for me like nobody else. In fact, before I left, on his recommendation alone, I was cast in a small budget independent film as a sports commentator for a triathlon featuring morbidly obese "athletes." When the director learned of my return trip to Oklahoma, he arranged for the production company to fly me back to California for the shoot. *I was going to be in a movie!*

The filmmaker's vision was something I went right along with, even though I was secretly embarrassed and ashamed by my role. One of my supposed to be funny lines was: *"Just as a NASCAR crowd expects to see a crash, the crowd here today is secretly hoping that someone will clutch their chest and fall to the ground before this competition is over."* It was horrible. And as interesting as watching a straight to DVD release might have been, I'm kind of relieved that the film never saw the light of day.

Unfortunately, somewhere on a shelf, sits footage of a 500-pound Sean, basically making fun of even bigger guys as they competed in this ill-conceived competition. I see the so-called "comedy" they were going for, but I can't help but to feel bad for everyone of those big guys who were submitting themselves and accepting this kind of treatment and humiliation, for the sake of "being in a movie." It was an acceptance I no longer wanted in my life. I wonder how many of those actors were feeling the same emotions. *I wonder how many are no longer with us?*

While I was waiting for a connecting flight on the way home, my cell phone rang again with a familiar area code. I was in a food court at DFW Airport, stuffing my face with Taco Bell. I wiped the sauce from my lips as I answered the call. It was a Jimmy Kimmel Live producer, asking if I were available. I was short in my answer, just a very simple, *"No, I'm not."* I didn't try to figure out how I could do it, I didn't ask any questions about the specifics of the bit, because it didn't matter. I no longer was a part of that scene. I was a thirty-minute flight and a ninety-minute drive away from my family and a new start in Ponca City. There was a peace coming over me, a back-to-basics attitude with the well-being of my family as the number one concern, not the pursuit of my comedy dream. Even though it sometimes felt like comedy success was knocking on my Los Angeles door, I now realized that real success for me was waiting back home in Oklahoma.

Because really, I *wasn't* pursuing my dream in comedy. I was constantly pursuing, chasing, *becoming addicted* to the acceptance I felt when everyone was laughing. I've drawn this conclusion, simply because of the lengths I would go to be something I was never honestly comfortable with in the first place.

I had been a morbidly obese person for so long that I began to celebrate my condition, accepting myself, even if it meant an early death. That horrible option was certainly much easier than actually doing something about changing. And I obviously didn't love myself enough to change, even though I would argue that I did love myself to a certain degree. But like an unhealthy love, it was an enabling one. I needed some tough love. And if tough love is hard to accept from others, it's twenty times harder to accept from ourselves, and accepting what I really needed would mean getting really honest about my behaviors with food. I wasn't ready. I was ready to focus on anything other than the revelations and admissions that might set me free. I needed a U-Haul truck because a new chapter of our lives was about to begin and everything was going to be just fine. I carefully loaded my fragile family and headed to Ponca City. Really, *this is just what we needed.*

Section Four

Stability at Last...for a Time

"I begin to see the truth of my addiction."

Chapter Twenty-Two

Living Large

Moving into a small two-bedroom apartment took some adjusting. Irene cried the first time she walked into this little place, but it didn't take long for her to make it uniquely ours. I didn't care how small it was, and eventually Irene felt the same way. The most important thing was that we were all together. Amber was starting eighth grade and Courtney fifth, I was starting my fifth round of employment with Team Radio, and Irene was looking for a job. We were a family on the move, filled with positive energy and hope.

Within six months we were ready to buy our first home. It was one of the most exciting experiences of our lives. After renting for so long, the feeling of ownership gave us pride and an increased sense of well-being. We were getting stronger than ever. Our financial troubles were subsiding thanks to our dual income and our stress level was at an all-time low. I had always said how easy it would be to lose weight if I could just be relieved of the daily stress that seemed to keep me running to food. Now, everything was brand new, we had reformed our family and restructured our lives in most every way. It was finally time to lose weight. All of the factors were in place for our success. We just had to start. A short two months after we closed on the house, we embarked on a family weight loss plan that would complete the transformation of our life and family. At least that was the plan.

Waiting for everything to be perfect before trying to lose weight is a serious problem because it works wonderfully as long as everything is perfect. This "perfect time" mentality was setting us up for a harsh reality down the road, when we would realize that there can't be a substitute for dealing with our issues, in the midst of a sometimes chaotic life. But, with everything as perfect as it could be, we joyously walked every night, all four of us. We ate dinner together nearly every night and all of us had a calorie budget we were managing. It sounds very familiar, but believe me, *it isn't.*

The weight was falling off with our consistent effort, but a crucial element was missing for me. I really hadn't come to terms with my food addiction. I couldn't bring myself to admit my addiction, so I wandered aimlessly down the road, lusting for food and fighting it all the way. I was looking for any excuse to cut loose and eat whatever I wanted. I made losing the weight a horrible chore because I hated the smaller portions. I hated not drinking regular Coke. I was losing weight simply because I was eating less and exercising every night. I wasn't making any real mental changes because—*why should I?* I didn't have a problem and I was doing what I needed to do to lose the weight, right? Sure, of course, I was. As long as everything remained semi-perfect, keeping the stress level low, the bills paid—*I could do this.* I could lose this weight once and for all. *I was on my way.*

We started on March 15th, 2004, and by July I had lost over one hundred pounds. Irene and the girls had also lost an incredible amount of weight and we were all feeling like a million bucks. At just under 400 pounds, I was feeling lighter than I had in years. I felt like I even looked small, compared to my 500-pound self, which is exactly what I weighed on March 15th.

I stepped on the scale July 20th, 2004 and found 397 in front of me. I had successfully, for the first time in my life, lost over one hundred pounds. It was time to celebrate, and since it was also Courtney's eleventh birthday, the celebration was already planned at The Hideaway.

I had lost one hundred three pounds in just over four months. I had earned an all-out celebration feast, or at least that's what I told myself.

In retrospect, it was like an alcoholic celebrating sobriety with a drink. The fried mushrooms were my favorite, and they still are my favorite. On that day, I announced to the family that I was ordering an extra order of mushrooms all to myself. I was giving everyone fair warning. This big bowl of fried mushrooms was all mine. Don't even think about it Courtney, not even on your birthday.

The pizza and fried mushroom feast was monumental. Everyone had their fill and I had enough to fill several people. I was justified in my gorging because I had worked hard to lose 103 pounds. Oh, sure, I still had a ways to go, but I wasn't worrying about it that day. I was finally free. Not free from obesity, but free from the restrictive calorie budget that I focused on for over one hundred and twenty days.

No problem, I would just get back on the wagon tomorrow, right? As we all posed for a family photo afterward, I somehow realized that something had changed. I was smaller and that was good. But like a shark tasting blood, I was frenzied in my day of devouring the portion sizes that I had avoided. I calmly tried to convince myself that this was just a temporary diversion, a pit stop along my transformation road, and that I would somehow snap back the next day. But there wasn't any snapping back. Like my ninety-nine-cent chicken fried steak meltdown at fourteen years old, I was completely back to my old behaviors. Although it would take me a month or so to really admit the truth.

Suddenly, it was much easier to make an excuse for why we didn't have time to walk every night. But still, we all pretended to be "on plan." I started sneak eating again, hiding my consumption from Irene and the girls and everyone at the radio station. There was hardly a day that someone didn't compliment me on my weight loss success, but what they didn't know was, in the privacy of my vehicle, I was consuming hundreds and probably thousands of calories in fast food escapes. I was spiraling out of control and I knew it, but felt powerless to change the course.

A couple of weeks after that infamous celebration feast day, we were doing something we hadn't enjoyed in a few years. We were going on vacation! The last vacation we took was a working vacation, where I worked the comedy clubs in Amarillo, Albuquerque, and Tuscon, while Irene and the girls stayed at the hotel. It was the only way we could afford a trip and every cent I earned paid for our lodging and other expenses. This vacation was going to be different. No comedy clubs, just family fun in Kansas City watching the Royals play baseball and enjoying Worlds of Fun amusement park. But something else was different.

We were still half-way pretending that all of us was still going strong on our family weight loss mission. I somehow managed to lose another twelve pounds, bringing my total 2004 weight loss to 115 pounds. If the feast at The Hideaway didn't completely crash my weight loss momentum, this upcoming vacation would surely do the trick.

None of us wanted to voice our concerns about our vacation food plan. Everyone was thinking about it, but no one dared to suggest or admit that we were completely off the wagon. As we drove out of town, there was a tension in the vehicle. How would we handle eating out on vacation and still stick to our calorie budgets? The truth was, I hadn't been sticking with the plan since the pizza and mushroom celebration, but Irene and the girls didn't know. We weren't ten miles down the highway when I decided to relieve the unspoken tension with a simple announcement:

"Girls, I have an idea. We're on vacation, so we're not going to worry about counting calories for the next four days. Let's just have fun and enjoy ourselves, and someone, please pass me a Nutty Bar." Everyone excitedly agreed and since JoEllen, Irene's sister, had supplied us with a sack full of road snacks, it took all of a few seconds for us to start digging in and taking advantage of the announced calorie relief proposal. The tension was gone, replaced with a joyful

celebration of our adventure ahead and an urgency to load up on some good food!

Just South of Wichita, only an hour into our trip, we stopped at a McDonald's. It was the first of many meals along this trip, where excess was celebrated and calorie budgets and exercise were dirty words. I remember ordering a Double Quarter-Pounder with Cheese and a Filet-O-Fish. Oh, yeah, this was my favorite McDonald's meal, complimented with fries and a real big *real* Coke. Oh, yeah, I knew exactly how to be careless and unlimited in my calorie consumption. This was just me, being me. The limits that had put me below 400 pounds for the first time since my teen years was just a forced existence, completely unnatural and completely void of the self-honesty about my food addiction and compulsive eating tendencies.

As soon as we arrived in Overland Park, an affluent suburb of Kansas City, we checked into our hotel and discovered something that excited us all. This hotel had a free eat-all-you-can deluxe continental breakfast, and that was perfect for our three-night stay. We were determined to make this hotel rethink its free breakfast strategy, and we did, but first we needed to unload and find a buffet restaurant somewhere.

Hometown Buffet was perfect for our second lunch, or early dinner, or whatever you want to call it. Obsession, maybe? We took full advantage of the buffet with a glorious disregard for calories or any sense of normal. I was leading my family down a detour without the possibility of getting back on the road we deeply desired and needed. We were lost and perfectly happy with the situation. Not wasting any opportunity to gorge, we even ordered late night pizza, delivered straight to our room at nearly midnight. It's very sad to me now as I recall the events, but at the time, we were happier than we had been in some time. The comfort, convenience, and carelessness of our vacation dining left us fat and happy and completely void of even a shred of the commitment we exhibited over the previous four months.

I planned on buying some new jeans on this trip and still, at nearly 400 pounds, the Big and Tall store was my only option. Or so I thought. I bought some size fifty Levi's, two pairs, for nearly seventy dollars. Coming from a size sixty-four, these new jeans were small. I was thrilled, but not as much as I would be about a half hour later.

On the way back to the hotel, Irene spotted a thrift store in a strip mall. She snapped, "Stop!" I was frustrated because I was in a hurry to get back to the hotel to try on my new jeans. Irene insisted on stopping, so I did. I waited in the vehicle while she and the girls shopped. After nearly twenty minutes, my frustration level was nearing its limit. I didn't want to spend my vacation in a strip mall parking lot. I charged into the thrift store and like a complete jerk, I loudly questioned Irene, *"What's taking you so long?"* Her reply left me feeling like the worst husband and father in the world. *"I found you some jeans in your size. They're nearly new, and cost only four bucks all together, for both pair!"* I was speechless. They didn't buy a single thing for themselves, just me, and imagine that—jeans from a store that wasn't a Big and Tall? This was exciting to me in the best way. My weight loss success up to that point was starting to show me changes that thrilled.

We hurried back to the hotel and after trying on the size fifty thrift store jeans, we decided to return the expensive Levi's for a full refund. These new jeans filled me with confidence like never before. I looked slimmer wearing those things. I was on top of the world and as we headed to Kaufman Stadium that evening, I was experiencing a mix of emotions. I was excited about these new jeans, but at the same time, I felt ultimately doomed from the old food behaviors that I allowed to come roaring back into my life. Oh, well, maybe some ballpark food would cheer me up!

The Royals radio network was trying to sign the sports station in the Team Radio family of stations, so it only took a call to secure an exclusive behind the scenes VIP tour of the stadium before the game. We felt like celebrities, chatting with major league players in the dugout and standing behind home plate during batting practice. We were the envy of the crowd in the stands, leaving them to wonder who we were and why we were allowed to mingle among the players. It was very special and along with my newly acquired size fifties, I was feeling euphorically confident and happy.

By the time the most amazing fireworks display signaled the end of an amazing night at the ballpark, we had consumed nachos, hotdogs, pretzels, and an ice cream shake. They actually had ice cream shake vendors walking the stadium steps and shouting, *"Get your creamy cold delicious ice cream shakes heeeerrrrreeeee!"* This was heaven to me. Sitting in a world-class major league stadium with my family and having ice cream shakes delivered right to my seat. A seat that, despite my lower weight, was still a very snug fit, but still possible—something I couldn't have done at 500 pounds.

At the Kansas City Zoo the next day, our trek was fairly easy. A hundred pounds lighter than when we made our Tulsa Zoo visit nine years previous, this time was drastically different, enjoyable for a change. I had every reason to celebrate and every reason to hold tight to the fundamentals that had brought me this far. I was wearing some awesome jeans, I was able to walk around an entire zoo without too much trouble, I was feeling wonderfully confident in my smaller size, and after nearly losing everything important to me, I once again was surrounded by the loving adoration of my beautiful family. Life was good and seemingly poised to get even better.

Worlds of Fun was another opportunity to experience life a hundred pounds lighter. I still couldn't fit on everything, but I did squeeze onto the ship ride, the log ride, and a water coaster that was designed in such a fashion that I could fit even at over 500 pounds. This was just a taste of how life could be if I kept on losing weight. A bit more enjoyable, but still, I felt severely restricted by my nearly four-hundred-pound body. I wouldn't fully enjoy a theme park until the fall of 2009, but that's later in the story.

Unfortunately, my food addiction and compulsive eating behaviors would quickly return me and, with my leadership, my family, back into a familiar existence. When the trip was over, so was any semblance of our plan. Our new habits and routine, completely replaced with the line of least resistance, where *"we really need to get back to walking and counting calories,"* could be heard every so often, before fading entirely into a distant memory of a weight loss dream we once shared.

Chapter Twenty-Three

511 and Holding

As the weight reclaimed my temporary taste of freedom, other wonderful opportunities presented themselves. In September of 2004, I was "hired" to perform stand-up on a bus trip from Vegas to Pasadena for OSU's football season opener with UCLA. The trip was with Triple Play Sports Radio, a part of the company I called home, and it included a flight to Vegas! I hadn't been on a plane in years, and even though nearly fifty pounds was already back on me, I was still feeling and looking smaller than my previous 500-pound weight.

The airplane seat was really small, but somehow I squeezed into it and fastened the extension belt. I reminded myself that it wouldn't have been much of a positive experience at my heaviest, but seriously, those thoughts did nothing to jolt me back to reality. I was once again fully engulfed in and embracing my obesity. My job on this trip was making people laugh with my brutal brand of self-deprecating material. This time, I was uniquely performing on a chartered bus traveling at seventy miles per hour through the same Mojave Desert where I experienced the slow and steady clarity that rightfully sent me packing from my Los Angeles home just a year and a half prior. The sad irony wasn't lost on me. The people laughed and I was getting paid. There I was, once again being the best fat guy I knew how to be. Big-fat-fun Sean, pretending to enjoy myself, as I hopelessly fell right back into being the lovable yet miserable 500-pound man I had been for so many years.

On the blackjack tables of The Golden Nugget, I had two goals: Win money and get as many food comps as possible. I managed to do both surprisingly well. I won a few hundred bucks and over the course of our three-day stay, I charmed my way into a seafood buffet comp and a complete, whatever you want, as much as you want, breakfast comp for three. The only thing better than all of the good food in Vegas is getting that food for free! I was completely out of control and raging right back to my previous existence.

Upon my return, the weight continued to pile back. I could no longer fit into my smaller jeans and soon I was right back in my size sixty-fours. I honestly believed that I would never again need these giant jeans, except to show them off in a classic weight loss "after" photo. My clothes had switched places. The smaller jeans and shirts made an undisturbed home in our closet, while the 500-pound wardrobe was back in business, one hundred percent.

I noticed that, not only did my friends and family sympathize with me over my weight gain, I did too. I excused my behaviors and weight gain by mentioning how hard it was to keep off and everyone agreed. I wasn't feeling too bad about it all because *this* is what happens. This was hard work and regaining was just an accepted part. I was the victim. *Poor me.*

I would speak of my weight gain like it was some kind of uncontrollable scientific proof that couldn't be avoided. Whatever I needed to tell myself and others to make it all better, that's what I did. It was a shame. A good start, completely destroyed by my inability to get real about my addiction and compulsions with food. My avoidance of self-responsibility was a perfect companion to this victim mentality. Going all the way back to 500 pounds and more was unavoidable because I never fully recognized and accepted my issues. I focused solely on the mechanics of weight loss, completely ignoring the emotional and psychological issues that cannot be ignored for real success.

Simply put, I didn't want to change my lifestyle or relationship with food because to me it wasn't necessary. I changed my day-to-day habits temporarily for those temporary results, and since the changes were just superficial, everything came back as soon as I gave up the charade and returned to being me. It's amazing to me now, how I couldn't see the flaws that would eventually wipe away that success. I was smug, I was confident, I knew it all, but somehow, I didn't know that my inability to be honest with myself would poison and kill every effort for self-improvement.

With my regaining, my lymphedema issues became worse. My right leg was in constant need of care, and Irene would again save me time and time again. When I would get lazy and choose to ignore the situation, the sores would eventually get so bad, they couldn't be ignored. The pain became too much to handle. Like clock-work, about every six months, I would need to take off a week at a time for healing. When the healing time started growing to a week and a half, Bill grew increasingly frustrated with the medical leave request.

Bill's frustration was much like Irene's in a way. They both could see that I was accepting this existence, and doing absolutely nothing to change. Irene would always be my caregiver and Bill would always allow me the paid time off to get well. That was the unspoken attitude that my actions, or inaction, projected. Eventually, Irene would voice her opinion about this very attitude and after several medical leave requests, Bill was finally reaching his limit.

After requesting yet another "healing time," Bill called me into his office for a tough talk. He told me that I had to do something about my weight and that he was becoming exhausted with my chronic absences. He suggested that I look into weight loss surgery. This was a last resort and one that actually sounded good to me because I felt so far away from ever grabbing control. My order from Bill was simple: Call and discuss a possible surgery with the company medical insurance plan.

I made that call fully expecting the insurance company to support and encourage the decision. Didn't it make sense to pay for a surgery now and avoid bigger problems and charges later? But for some reason, the insurance company didn't think that way. I was told that they wouldn't cover the cost and since there was no way we could afford the surgery, it suddenly wasn't an option. I honestly didn't want the surgery because I was convinced that I knew how to lose weight, if I wanted. And I did know the basic formula for weight loss, eat less and exercise, but I didn't know that those elements were a small fraction of the overall dynamics needed for lasting success.

If I was going to lose weight, I had to do it on my own, and that was a scary idea. I was back up to over 500 pounds and feeling as hopeless as ever. Instead of really doing something about the situation, I simply ignored it, trying to not complain or ask for too much time off.

Irene was still wrapping me every day with low-stretch compression bandages, as we tried frantically to keep the swelling in check enough to avoid skin breakage. It was easy for me. All I had to do was roll the wraps and sit there while Irene did all the work. And as much as Irene loved me and did this because of that love and devotion, she was growing very tired of my total acceptance of the situation. Knowing that weight loss could possibly improve this situation dramatically, and never seeing me have even an ounce of weight loss motivation and commitment, took its toll on Irene's attitude. I couldn't blame her. I was seriously taking advantage of her.

My weight was getting much harder to handle. Every year seemed to be a little harder than before. The intimacy within our marriage became non-existent. I was so completely repulsed by myself, I didn't have the desire to be intimate. I didn't even want to touch me, let alone my wife of twenty years. Our marriage became a caregiver-patient relationship. The intimacy was completely gone, save for a goodbye kiss and an "I love you" every day.

Part of my refusal to deal with my weight issues included refusing to fully acknowledge the damage it was doing to our marriage and family. It was killing me and our marriage, or more specifically—I was killing me and my family in a slow, painful fashion. The days turned into weeks and the weeks into months, and before long I was looking back on four years since I lost the 115 pounds in 2004.

I somehow managed to "maintain" right around 500 pounds. I have no idea how, considering that I wasn't trying to watch anything. It's like my body had a set limit for gaining. The highest weight I remember seeing was 511 pounds. I guess I was lucky to have this mysterious "gaining limit" because it allowed me to get by without being completely incapacitated.

When I was asked to perform stand-up the first Friday in June of 2008, I happily accepted. I was opening for the Beatles tribute band, 1964 at a big concert following a huge community event called "Draggin' Grand." Even though my weight "maintained" right around five hundred or just slightly over, it was becoming much harder to handle. Even though I once moved about the stage at five hundred with relative ease, this performance was noticeably different.

I couldn't breathe. I couldn't move. My style was mic in hand, roaming the stage, but this performance was so exhausting, I just left the mic in the stand and stood in one place. The comedy bits that required physical movement were modified because, if I tried to be as animated as before, I wouldn't be able to catch my breath. It was the longest thirty minutes of my stand-up career. Never before did I feel so labored just standing in one place speaking. Despite the labored and obviously difficult set, the audience was laughing, and several complimented my routine afterward. But I knew something had seriously changed. My weight might not have been going up much past five hundred, but my body's tolerance was wearing thin, and was about to reach a breaking point.

In the days after that stand-up performance, my breathing became much worse and the occasional pains in my chest became more frequent. Something felt horribly wrong and I was starting to once again become frightened with the thought that my "someday" was going to be a little too late. I felt like I was walking a tight rope and I could fall to my death at any moment. In the early morning hours of June 10th, I made the decision to call Gayle Williams in to do my radio show so that I could go to the doctor.

Chapter Twenty-Four

The End . . . Again

I normally avoided the doctor because I knew exactly what was coming. I had heard it countless times in the past. I needed to lose weight and find a way to keep it off. Blah, blah, blah, blah . . . I understand! But as much as I avoided the doctor, I knew that I couldn't avoid it this time. Like a prisoner finding religion, I fully embraced the hope of a doctor's help, fueled by desperation and fear, as I made my way into the office.

"What brings you in today?" It was an expected question, but I didn't have an answer really; I just knew something wasn't right. *"I don't know, I just need checked. I don't feel right."* I was teetering on an emotional breakdown and the receptionist could tell, I'm sure. I was scared. Given my emotional state, it didn't take much for the doctor to push me over the edge.

The doctor, she could sense my fear and emotion, and she knew it was the perfect opportunity to maybe make an impact with her professional assessment. When she discovered my blood pressure was 220/119, she absolutely unleashed the horrible truth that I had tried to avoid for so long. She told me that if I were a pregnant woman, I would be immediately taken to the hospital for an emergency C-section. My blood pressure was killing me, pure and simple. As she described the impact my blood pressure and obesity was having on my internal organs, I was completely reduced to tears. It was as if she was giving me an inescapable death sentence, an inevitable fate that was waiting to kill and wreak havoc in the lives of my loved ones. She topped her speech with this: If you leave our office today and drop dead walking across the parking lot, none of us in here would be the least bit surprised.

I was shaken, in tears, and afraid of every breath—thinking it might be my last. For the first time in a very long time, I didn't want to run to food for comfort. I wanted to live and that meant immediately making the changes and choices that could possibly save my life. I survived the walk to the van, and I sat there and sobbed. I felt alone and scared, so I called Irene and explained what was happening. I promised her that this was it, I was starting right this second. I wasn't waiting until "someday," or until Monday, or until some future, more perfect starting date. I was starting *now*.

I arrived home and found Irene and the girls waiting for me in the driveway. My face was red and wet and so were theirs. I climbed out of the van and we all embraced and wept. I felt so loved and so clear about what I had to do. I had a choice. Live or die. It was that black and white. I wanted to live and whatever that meant I needed to do, that was what I would do. As I looked into the tear-filled eyes of my wife and kids, I made them a promise, this time would be different. Unfortunately, it didn't take long for us to realize that my food addiction and emotional eating compulsions were far stronger than my commitment to change, even in the face of a certain early death.

I quickly filled my blood pressure medicine prescription and started counting every single calorie. I had to do this, for real. My commitment lasted for two and a half days. It's very hard to understand the rationale that goes into a meltdown in the face of overwhelming emotion and desperate purpose. I've tried to figure it out and it's one of the most challenging dynamics.

Maybe I was given an out because this new blood pressure medicine would save me, instead of me saving me. The stress and pressure to do what I needed to do was too much to handle. When I added the personal financial stress that we were experiencing, including facing possible foreclosure, well—I was left running to the only place I knew to find comfort, peace, and shelter from the storm of stress.

This wasn't a good time for me to try to lose weight. If the blood pressure medicine could buy me a little more time, maybe we could reach a point where life wasn't so stressful. I always proclaimed that the only thing holding me back from weight loss success was daily stress. I'm a stress eater, so I was in serious trouble. Now, more than ever, my weight was causing me a mountain of additional stress, and that made it even harder to get a handle on anything.

By late afternoon on June 12th, 2008, I was headed into the neighborhood grocery store to buy ice cream. Blue Bell was on sale and it was my favorite, Moolinium Crunch. I quietly grabbed the half-gallon from the freezer and made my way to the checkout. I paid the five bucks and made my way three blocks to the safe confines of my home. I walked in, grabbed a spoon, and plopped onto the couch, channel surfing and comforting myself with every creamy delicious bite. This was the end.

I have no way of knowing what Irene, Courtney, and Amber were thinking when they witnessed this obvious relapse. But judging from the disappointed looks, they were equally confused and saddened by this sudden turn. I wasn't really enjoying the ice cream that day, I was medicating my emotions. I was curbing my stress with a pleasurable experience. I was addicted to the escape the ice cream provided. I wasn't worried about my blood pressure, my swollen lymphedema-stricken right leg, my strained relationship with my employer, or the fact that we were severely behind on our mortgage. None of that mattered while I was getting lost in that half-gallon. It was my one-way ticket away from the reality that was suffocating. When I had my fill, I put the remainder in the freezer, and looked for a comfortable place to take a late afternoon nap. Eating and sleeping, as much as possible, both provided the temporary escape from the honest truth that threatened to take me and my family down. Two things that could have been so good, an ice cream treat and good sleep, were instead used and abused. They became some of the tools of my self-destruction.

There was no such thing as getting back on the wagon the next day, not after a meltdown like this, oh, no. It would be weeks, maybe months, before inspiration or what was thought to be a near death experience would jolt me back to a starting point. Up until this point, nothing worked. I had tasted weight loss freedom back in 2004, and it wasn't enough. I had been given what seemed like a death sentence from my doctor several times, and it wasn't enough. I had endured the painful sores on my leg, all the while knowing that weight loss might not fix it, but would certainly improve the situation dramatically, but still, it wasn't enough of a motivator.

The stress of life was raining down, and more honestly, the stress from the consequences of our horrible choices in managing our finances, was keeping me far away from worrying about my weight. In the months after that June doctor's visit, weight loss start, then fail, we lost our home to the bank and had to move into a rental, and we were sending Amber off to college without a shred of financial support.

This was not how it was supposed to be, *what kind of parents were we?* We had more bills than income, creating a constant source of stress that strained everything in our lives. This wasn't the time to think about weight loss. All of our energy was focused on surviving, coping with the situation we had created. For me, that meant finding as much comfort and peace in food as possible. It's all I had ever known. It's what I did, and short of winning the lottery, it wasn't about to change anytime soon, *or was it?*

Section Five

Steel Curtain Zone

"I finally learn it is my choice to be a victim or champion."

Chapter Twenty-Five

Last Chance Exit

The one thing I always had was the love and understanding from my family. The love that surrounded me as a child and the love given me by my young family was something I cherished. When Irene and I were separated years prior, it ripped me apart, and left me scrambling to get us back together. Now, we were back together, a strong family bond that, despite everything else, was always there. And I really thought it would always be there. At least I did until the night of September 13th, 2008.

We were in the tiny town of Thomas, Oklahoma, staying the night with the Eakins, Amber's boyfriend's parents. Amber was just starting her freshman year at Southwestern Oklahoma State University and we were there for a family day on campus. I don't remember much about the day and the events leading up to that night, but something was brewing inside Irene. It had been building for years, and as if she was unable to control or contain her emotions, she let it all out right there in the guest room of the Eakins household.

"I'm done." Two simple little words. That's what she said. I didn't know what she meant, I thought she was just exhausted from the day, ready for bed. I had no idea of what was about to come from her lips.

"I'm done watching you kill yourself. I love you, I do, but I can't stand by and witness your slow suicide any longer. I want a divorce." Her words were filled with several different emotions. Anger, love, hopelessness, fear, desperation, and she was serious, I could see it in

her eyes. Never before do I remember seeing such a look from her. This was serious and it didn't matter that we were a guest in someone's home that night.

I immediately tried to make her feel bad about what she was saying. *"So, we get one off to college and you can't hold it together long enough for us to get the other one out of high school? How could you do this to Courtney? Can't we talk about this later, why now, why here?"* And as she collapsed on the bed, crying, I knew that she had reached her limit. It didn't matter where we were or what we were doing. It was like she had no control over this release of emotion. Maybe it was her last ditch effort to snap me back into reality. Maybe she loved me enough to walk away, thinking that it might spark the changes I needed to save my own life.

It didn't take me long to realize that I was wrong in what I was saying and doing in that moment. This wasn't her fault, and she couldn't help it; she had reached her emotional capacity. That's when I started to negotiate with her, begging for one more chance to turn it all around. She had heard it all before, why should she believe me now? But just as I had never witnessed that look in her eyes, she must have noticed the same difference in my frantic proposal. Because she was listening to me. This was my chance to promise her one last time. I owed it to her, my daughters, and I really owed it to myself to make a change once and for all. This was it.

I asked for a day to get my plan together and figure out how I was going to make this happen, and on Monday September 15th, 2008, I would start. *"This time is going to be very different,"* I pleaded. *"It's got to be, buddy, it's got to be."* And with those words from her, we embraced and cried, cleansing our emotions and sending us to sleep with a relief, different for each of us. Her rest was made better because she released all of the emotions that had been building for so long and I rested because I dodged a bullet that night. But now, the real challenge would start and I didn't have any room for failure. I had to get it right. Sunday the fourteenth was spent contemplating how I was going to make this time different from every other weight loss attempt. My family depended on it, and so did my life, but obviously I was more scared of losing my family than I was my life. I know that doesn't really make sense, but it does when you really think about the mental dynamics.

Dying young was something tragic that happened to other people. I was a survivor, remember? Every time my obesity would make me fear for my life, I would cling to something that would make me feel better about it all. *Oh, so it's not a heart attack, just indigestion? Or, it's out of control blood pressure, but that can be treated, right?* I always found the outs, I always found the thoughts or the solutions that would let me off the hook and make me feel better about my inaction in confronting the real issues. My weight was killing me and now it was killing my family. And there wasn't anything I could do or say that would make it all better, unless it was exactly what I needed, and that meant getting to the bottom of my issues with food and once and for all, losing the weight.

Waking up on Monday September 15th, 2008, was very different. This was my Day One. As I laid there staring up at the ceiling, I thought about how this was *the day*. It was very different because many times I would start by completely forgetting that I had planned to "start." It was typical for me to realize what I was supposed to do, only after the sugar of my morning Coke hit my tongue. Another false start because I would have already "ruined" the attempt. Oh, well, maybe next time, *bring on the fried cinnamon roll!* Not this time. It was so powerful, on the top of my brain, it was an all-consuming thought as soon as my eyes opened that morning.

I honestly felt like this was my last chance. The changes that would come if I failed were too horrible. I would lose my family as I knew it and die young. I had to grab control and choose the change. I had to keep it together and be consistent like never before. *But how? H*ow would this time be different? I honestly didn't know the answer, but I decided that it would work itself out along the way. I knew that I had to constantly remind myself to stay on track and if I could successfully keep myself from blowing it, then maybe I could finally break free. The focus wasn't on the food, it was squarely on the mental dynamics, I was walking a tight rope, where it didn't matter how I stayed balanced—as long as I didn't fall. It was the beginning of, what I would later realize and appropriately name, my "Steel Curtain Zone."

Chapter Twenty-Six

Choosing Change

W hat I was facing had to be on the most honest level possible. I was a food addict. I had never honestly acknowledged that fact at the beginning of a weight loss attempt, but I did this time. I knew that I depended on food in every way. I was a stress eater, an emotional eater, a happy eater, a celebratory eater, everything revolved around food, always. Changing that dependency was paramount to my success. Could I somehow survive without the crutch of food supporting every emotion? The answer was yes, but it wasn't going to be easy. *Or was it?*

I was always conditioned to believe that weight loss had to be hard. How many times have you heard someone say, *"losing weight is so hard!"* That was me. And I always would follow that statement with a long list of reasons why I probably couldn't succeed. My biggest excuse was always stress. *"I'm under too much stress, and when I'm stressed, I eat. That's just the way it is, so I guess I'm just out of luck. No weight loss for me!"*

If this time was going to be different, I had to convince myself that it didn't have to be hard. I had to believe that I could succeed. And I had to take it one day at a time, often, one hour at a time. My goal that day and every day was simple: Make it to the pillow tonight, knowing that I stayed within the bounds of my calorie budget and with some kind of exercise on the books. I was simplifying the start-up. Fifteen hundred calories and walking as far as I could handle, that was the plan on Day One. It didn't matter what I decided to eat, it could be anything, as long as it was within my budget. I was treating my calories like cash, thus starting what I would eventually refer to as my "Calorie Bank and Trust."

Treating the calories like cash simplified the process. I wasn't devoting all of my energies to food list or grocery shopping trips, picking up items I would never eat "in real life." I wasn't the least bit concerned about fat grams, or sodium, or anything other than the almighty calorie. The calorie was my currency, and this different way of looking at my calorie budget made it all seem fun and challenging. Every morning I would wake up and an imaginary teller would hand me fifteen hundred calories to spend however I wanted. The only catch? When they're gone, *they're gone*. If I blew them all early in the day, it would be a very long wait until the next day's allowance. Because the Calorie Bank and Trust doesn't have an ATM, or over-draft protection, or a loan department.

Gone were the rationalizations that excused bad choices. *Well, I'm going to eat more tonight, but I'll eat less tomorrow,* or *I'll work out extra hard, then enjoy this giant ice cream shake,* or one of my favorites, *I've been so good lately, I deserve to cut loose and enjoy myself.* All of these and more usually started to surface in past weight loss attempts, infecting my resolve, breaking me down, and eventually ending the attempt. The more I would write about these thoughts and mental dynamics, the more I started to understand the absurdity of it all. That's why I don't believe in "cheat days."

Allowing one day to just go completely nuts and gorge is a food addict's way of dealing with a restrictive calorie budget. If I can look forward to that day, then maybe I can keep it together, hold on, eat less, exercise more, and then—*oh, boy, watch out!* It's "reward feast" time. I repeatedly did just this, until this time. The self-honesty I was applying to my journey was shining a light on every element that I allowed to keep me from success before. And staying consistent while looking forward to cutting loose and eating as much as you desire shows just how temporary the changes can be. If my goal was to become a responsible eater and to redefine my relationship with food, then I didn't have a need to break away from my "restrictive diet" with a cheat day.

Chapter Twenty-Seven

No Pills, No Surgery, and No Salad

It was never about being restricted. That's why I've always touted "nothing is off limits" because this new relationship with food must include all foods, good and bad. I can't just avoid my issues with ice cream by saying, *"I'm not allowed to eat ice cream anymore."* I had to find a way to enjoy what I liked to eat in a new, more reasonable way. I've said it many times, *"I eat what I like and nothing I don't."* That's why I've never had a salad. I've tasted salad, on a dare, or as a trade to get Irene to try a bite of fish, or when my daughters asked me to, complete with a little cute frown-face (they know exactly how to get me to do almost anything. Just look sad when you ask, *"Daddy, will you please try my salad?"* Well, of course, as I hold my nose.

I use the salad as an example because I can't tell you how many times I've heard someone say, *"If you want to lose weight, you have to eat salads!"* It's just not true. If you want to lose weight, you have to eat normal portions of whatever you like, and exercise. Besides, I've laid eyes on some salads that contained double the calories of my entire meal, but it's a salad! As if, just because it's called a salad, it has magical weight loss properties. I could call a large deep dish pizza a salad, but eating it all will not help me lose weight. It all goes back to the self-honesty component.

Why was I always quick to excuse bad choices before? Because I was always my own worst enemy. Anything I could tell myself, any lie, to make myself feel better about bad choices, that's what I would do. It was a ridiculous cycle, a poison to every other weight loss attempt. And it's so easy because they start coming as a guise to being kind to ourselves. You've heard people say, *"Don't be so hard on yourself,"* and if I was trying to lose weight, I would cling to that, giving myself break after break, until I was fooling myself completely. Instead of being a friend, I was undermining and destroying every attempt, often before I could see any real results. And if I did see results, it would always come roaring back as soon as I returned to being me. This time, I wasn't just changing my behaviors with food, I was changing me, at my very core. The new behaviors and attitudes about food were really a side effect of my awakening. The Calorie Bank and Trust did things that I didn't even realize it would, helping me change my approach, and eventually leading me to freedom.

It forced me to make my food decisions based on calorie value. And it completely took the focus off the food and squarely where I knew it was needed on me and my tendency to allow anything and everything to send me running to the nearest convenience store deli, *or the bank.*

My bank was the greatest bank of all time. I'm talking about my actual bank, money, not calories. *Why were they the best banking institution in the free world?* Because every Monday and Friday it was cookie day. The tellers would bake up large batches of Otis Spunkmeyer Cookies, and even though you were supposed to come inside to get them, they knew me so well, they always shot them to me through the tube in the drive-thru. I would find a reason to go to the bank on Mondays or Fridays because I knew that fresh baked cookies were waiting my arrival.

"Uh, yeah, I just need you to check my balance, you know, just to see if I need to make a deposit or something." "Cookies?" "Well, I forgot it was Monday, lucky me! Of course, I would like one, or two, wow, three, thank you!" Soon, I didn't even need a reason. They would see me coming and quietly jet the cookies to my car. It was like some kind of drug deal, really. And my drug was white chocolate chip macadamia nut cookies.

Day One was cruising along just fine, and then, I had to go to the bank. Seriously, I really did. The fifteenth was payday. Before I could say anything, two freshly baked cookies came flying to me, just like always. This was a test. I didn't even take them out of the tube. I knew that if I did, they would probably find their way into my mouth, via my hands, and I couldn't do that this time. This time had to be different, remember? So I quickly pushed the "send" button, jetting them back to the stunned tellers. At first, I received an expression like, *that's the only kind we have today,* but mostly it was some kind of confusion among the tellers.

"Thank you, but I'm counting calories today, it's my Day One, and although I could have a cookie, I don't want to invest the calories." I remember a very friendly reply and a bunch of smiles. Smiles that said it all without saying a thing. I encountered those same smiles at work that day.

I can't blame my co-workers at the studio because I had said it many times, with different approaches, some with comical consequences. Everyone remembered my Vienna sausage, cheese, and pork skin diet, so I had some skeptical support from everyone around the station. But after the jokes about my past attempts, I could tell that everyone was hoping that this time would be different. But how was I going to make sure? I had lost 115 pounds in 2004 and gained it all back plus some, so what was going to be different this time?

Chapter Twenty-Eight

The Daily Diary of a Winning Loser

I was going to write about my feelings and experiences every night, a blog, that I would share with my friends and family on MySpace! That's how it would be different. But even better, this time I was admitting that I was seriously addicted to food and I needed some prayers, some strength, and some support from everyone in my world.

Before sitting down to write that Day One post, I gave some serious thought to content. I had to be brutally honest and open up about things that I would never have shared before. I never told people that I weighed over 500 pounds. If they guessed four hundred, so be it, they didn't need to know the truth. But just as I realized self-honesty with my choices was one of the most critical elements of my success, I also knew that honesty in my writing was just as important. *My daughters are going to read this,* I thought. My Day Two post was the first time I ever gave my true weight. It was exactly 505 pounds.

And really, my daughters reading this, was one of the biggest reasons I started my blog. I knew what I allowed morbid obesity to do to me and now I was passing those same habits and behaviors onto my daughters. We sent Amber off to college with over one hundred pounds to lose. Kids just follow the leaders in their life, and we were their leaders. We felt horrible guilt—so if I could share this journey with them, and it could help keep them inspired and motivated, well, that would be amazing to me and them.

Day One was hard to write, especially the part about daydreaming my own funeral. I did that all the time. I was always scared that today might be my last. I know it's true, no matter our physical condition, but at over 500 pounds, it seemed especially imminent and completely possible, just like the doctor said back in June. I could drop dead and nobody would question the reason or even wonder why, not even for a second. Then what? I would have that thought on a Sunday and think, *if that happens, my funeral would probably be on Thursday.* What a horrible thing to sit around and think about, but I did, all the time.

I didn't know how much I weighed on Day One because avoiding scales was a way of life. I knew that it had to be over 500 pounds, had to be, but I wasn't sure, maybe 510, 515? A trip to the scales was planned for Day Two. Yes, a trip. All the way to Stillwater, some forty-five miles to our South, my hometown, and the place where I had started many weight loss attempts: The Payne County Health Department. I couldn't find a scale to weigh me anywhere closer. Can you imagine? Seriously, not a scale in town, that I knew of, would do the trick. And I had to weigh, after all, many past attempts had been scrubbed because of me failing to get an accurate weight reading to start. Isn't that crazy? If I didn't know where I was starting, I couldn't start, or continue. I had to know! And this time was going to be very different.

I would often weigh and the only person in the entire world I would allow to know would be Irene. My mom? Forget it, I didn't want to worry her with my shocking number. Friends, family, co-workers? Not a chance. It was always a secret. But not this time, no— different, remember? This time it would be acknowledged on my newly formed blog for anyone to see. I was establishing a support system that required complete transparency.

I didn't really want to know myself, for I was scared. But at the same time, I was relieved that it wasn't higher than it was. Five hundred five. Wow, okay, here we go. *505 pounds.* The cool thing, I remember thinking, was that it wouldn't take long to break into the four hundreds! I was off and running! Well, uh, walking. Or whatever you want to call it, waddling? Sure, that's probably pretty accurate.

I knew that exercise had to be a major part of my efforts and walking was the only thing I could do at this point. Even walking had become a challenge. I would seriously become breathless just walking down a hallway at work, often answering the phone to a question: "Hey, are you going to be alright?"

Heading out to the walking trail was kind of scary to me. Courtney was by my side that first night. We pulled into the driveway of War Memorial Park and I immediately proclaimed the trail was too difficult. But we weren't leaving. Instead of walking around the trail, we decided to just walk around the perimeter of the actual Hutchins Memorial building. It was slow and painful. My feet were hurting to start, and even though it was a relatively cool September evening, I was sweating. I slowly wobbled around the building, making it once, before announcing that I was finished for the night. I did all I could do. Well, honestly, probably not "all I could do," but enough to feel threatened if I tried any more. I could feel some pain in my chest, my legs, and just about anywhere else on my body. Imagination was getting the best of me and in the name of safety, we headed to the vehicle feeling great about this momentous start. This time was different. I mean—it was much harder to do what I did before. Only four years separated my last major attempt from this time, but it felt like it had been twenty. All of a sudden, at thirty-six years old, my obesity was starting to take a serious toll on my body.

I wanted success this time, real, lasting, meaningful success. I really wanted to change. Not just physically, but mentally. I wanted to break myself from the addiction and emotional dependency I had with food my entire life. Slowly, one day at a time, one hour at a time, I was making it. Day One, Day Two, Day Three, this was becoming fun. Soon I was staring down my first weekend and that really made me nervous.

The work week was easier because I was kept busy most of the day. The weekend would give me more time to concentrate on doing well, and really, I was seriously afraid of that idle time. My iron-clad decision was made, I was doing this, so weekend or not, I was going to make it through. It just meant I would be battling myself a little more than I had before. More than ever before.

I decided that this was it, this was the time. It didn't matter the circumstances, the emotions, the stress, it just didn't matter. I could no longer let all of these outside forces dictate my behaviors with food. If I was really going to lose the weight once and for all, then I had to fight myself every time. With every urge or desire to overeat, I had to remind myself what I was doing and why I was doing it. I constantly kept my motivating thoughts fresh. If I was having a particularly tough time, I would often go to the bathroom and just look at my face in the mirror. Those internal conversations in my head were so important, especially in the beginning. And I wasn't just giving myself stern talks, I was also envisioning my future appearance. *What would I look like?* I had never lost enough to see that big of a change, even in 2004. *What would I look like at 230?* I couldn't even begin to imagine, I just had to stay with the plan. And the plan was to not really have a "plan."

I broke it down to the very basics as far as food and exercise were concerned. I could eat whatever I wanted as long as I didn't exceed fifteen hundred calories. The integrity of my Calorie Bank and Trust couldn't be broken, no matter what. That rule was set in stone. The exercise was all I could do, walk, walk, and walk some more. Deciding that failure wasn't an option this time really gave me a whole new approach. I almost expected to fail in the past. I just always knew that I was one stressful trigger away from a meltdown. I decided to throw away that line of thought. *It was bogus.*

That iron-clad decision forced me to deal with my everyday stress in other ways, and as long as I didn't break the bank, and as long as I exercised, I was winning, every day. I didn't even realize what I was doing in the beginning, but I was gradually evolving my good choices, simply because I was maneuvering through my calorie budget, trying to get the most bang for my calorie buck. I automatically started shunning high calorie choices, limiting my portions according to my budget, and noticing something very exciting.

I wasn't hungry. I wasn't! I was spreading my calories out as evenly as I wanted and I didn't feel deprived one iota. *Why?* Because I could have anything I wanted. *This is brilliant,* I thought. If nothing was off limits, then the only way to ever cheat was by breaking the bank, and that wasn't an option. It suddenly became impossible to cheat. Never again would I have a bite of something and declare, *"Well, I tried, and failed—I just had a half a Snickers bar, I messed up. Maybe I'll stick with it next time."* Nope, there wasn't a "next" time. This was *the time*—and if different was what I was aiming for, that's exactly what I was noticing. The big difference for me was the writing every night.

The blog was my lifeline, every night. It was a requirement. My writing was soul baring, but it also magnified where I was going right and where I had gone wrong for years. It was an introspective study, fueled by brutal self-honesty, and a very real epiphany that I had never realized.

My obesity? *It was my fault.* My behaviors with food? *They were all on me and nobody else.* It wasn't anyone or anything's fault. It wasn't the restaurant industry's fault, it wasn't because of my stressful finances, or the stress of raising teenage daughters. It wasn't my dad's fault for not being there for me when I was a kid and it wasn't my mother's fault for taking me to McDonald's. I was a grown man and I was in charge of my choices and I was choosing change before change chose me. Because change was coming.

Early death? Only God knows, but one thing is for sure. Just as I noticed the difference in four short years, as far as my mobility was concerned, at relatively the same weight, the changes coming would surely get worse from there. I was going to make one good choice after another, all the way to the finish. But wait, *finish?* No, there is no "finish." All the way for the rest of my life. I'm the captain—and I'll live or die by the consequences of my choices. And I'll have no one to blame but me, if I don't succeed.

I had never felt this empowered before. Everyone around me could see a change in my attitude. My step was lighter, and I faced everything with an attitude that oozed positive energy. It was having just the effect I had hoped. This joyous attitude for the process was very real and contagious, affecting those closest to me.

Amber was away at school, in her freshman year at Southwestern Oklahoma State University in Weatherford, and she was dropping weight, too. When everyone was dreading the "freshman 15," Amber was working out and losing four times that amount of weight. Courtney, Irene, and I would all eat dinner together and then we would all workout together. Courtney was dropping the weight, too, and Irene had already started dropping weight, even before I started. We were a shrinking family. It was an amazing time. Consistency was key in our success. And consistently writing the blog was also critical to my success. It was just as important as my nightly walking.

Chapter Twenty-Nine

Shifting Perspective

I was quickly learning the focus, the thing I looked forward to at family gatherings, didn't have to be on the food. It wasn't long into my journey when we hosted a backyard family cookout. *How would I navigate that?* It was easy because my focus wasn't on the food; it was on the loved ones around me. It had never been that way before. I could still enjoy a hamburger and a hotdog, maybe a few chips, save some calories by using half a bun, using mustard instead of mayo, little things to get the most out of my calorie budget. I would end up with a normal plate of food, and surprisingly, I was actually satisfied. *So this is how normal people approach food,* I thought. It was amazing to me, the difference in my enjoyment of the event. All of a sudden I was interested in the people I loved, instead of lusting after huge piles of food and half-listening to people as I ate everything.

I was always obsessed over the menu, and more than the menu, the quantity of food available, wherever we were. Instead of looking forward to the family visiting, I was looking forward to the nearly endless fried chicken. My approach, my attitude and perspective was rapidly changing. And so were the numbers on the scale.

I had decided to weigh every two weeks. I just decided. A bunch of people have asked me how or why I chose some of the variables along my road. *Why did you choose fifteen hundred calories? Why did you choose to weigh every two weeks?* The fifteen hundred calories seemed reasonable, since it was only five hundred calories less than the two thousand calorie recommended daily allowance. And the weighing every two weeks thing, well, that took a little more thought.

One of the things I realized about my past failed attempts was how I would create ways to feel discouraged. The biggest way to do this is to constantly weigh. I hadn't done it as an adult, really, because the scale was harder to find at my size. But I did when I was younger and smaller. Why would I want to do anything that might needlessly discourage? Our bodies fluctuate with fluid weight and weight from waste, and for all kinds of reasons. Allowing the scale to have power over my emotions just wasn't going to happen, unless those emotions were positive. Every two weeks was just perfect. I wasn't worried about what I would find on the scale. I understood that if I maintained the integrity of my calorie budget and I consistently exercised, then the positive results would come, with or without the scale, helping or hindering my emotions.

"No way, no way, can you believe that?" I was overwhelmed with happiness. Tears of joy filled Irene's eyes as I stepped onto the scale for that first two-week weigh-in. *"Twenty-one pounds in two weeks, wow, that's incredible. Four hundred eighty-four, I weigh four hundred eighty-four! Can you believe that?"* I had to have been one of the happiest 484-pound people in the world. It was unreal, really. I knew that a bunch of that had to have been water weight, but I also knew it wasn't all water. I was losing fat, too, and really, fat or fluid, I didn't care, as long as the number continued to drop. And drop it did. Weigh day after weigh day, every time, big losses. I was getting super spoiled. There was no stopping me now, and then Day Sixty came along and reminded me that I *wasn't* Superman.

Chapter Thirty

Life in the Danger Zone

Day Sixty was just one of those days when anything that could go wrong did. I was being tested at every turn. My stress level at work was very high, for whatever reason, and my financial stress was off the chart. I remember feeling like I was about to lose control. Keeping the lights on and gas in the vehicles were two things that were in jeopardy that day. Scrambling for a small loan to give us a temporary fix to our financial stress just added to my dwindling resolve. By the time I hit the door that afternoon, I didn't feel like working out and I didn't feel like caring about my calorie budget.

I was spent, completely. Gone was the joy that had brought me so far. Gone was my always positive attitude. I found a way to fix our immediate troubles, and now I was looking for an emotional fix. I stumbled out to the van and started driving, McDonald's sounded like the perfect poison. But I couldn't do it. I just couldn't pull the trigger on that binge. I wanted to really bad. I wanted to drown myself in a couple of double cheeseburgers and fries, and a Fillet-O-Fish, too, but I just couldn't make myself say the words needed to place the order.

"Take your time and let me know when you're ready." The McDonald's employee on the other end of that speaker had no idea of the emotional tug of war that was taking place in their drive-thru. I had come too far to throw it all away, and I knew that was exactly what would happen, if I allowed myself this meltdown. *What about that iron-clad decision I made? What about my motivating thoughts? What about my family?* They were so proud of me and my success, *how could I possibly let them down again? What would I tell the people that were reading my blog every day?*

"Sir, can I help you?" They were getting impatient with me. So I replied with an order. *"Give me a low-fat vanilla ice cream cone, please."* I had survived the moment with a one-hundred-fifty-calorie treat. I enjoyed the cone, but as I drove away the emotions of the day were trembling inside. I must have looked like the saddest man who ever licked a cone with Ronald's smiling face on the protective cone-sleeve, smiling back at my fragile face.

I had to get strong, I had to survive this day. All of a sudden I realized that my resolve to not let any emotion, circumstance, person, place, or thing steal this away from me was being tested. My Steel Curtain Zone was being tested! Even though I had survived the McDonald's drive-thru with a normal one-hundred-fifty-calorie treat, I wasn't out of the danger zone. I still had hours to go before bed. If I could somehow survive this day, I really thought, I could do this, this, meaning—I could really, once and for all, lose my weight, and become a normal-sized person. I was shaky at best, but I was winning, and I had to find cover, or, uh, *covers.* I didn't feel like writing the blog, but I had to do it; it was non-negotiable. So I did. And it was probably one of the shortest blog postings for me, ever.

I had to get to sleep. I had to get under the covers and shield my journey with pleasant unconsciousness. My escape was in dreamland, where I could put this horrible Day Sixty behind me and start with a new attitude for Day Sixty-One. That was absolutely the only way I was going to survive the day with my calorie budget in order. I had to go to bed, early, quickly, *now!*

Just as I had done the fifty-nine nights previous, I hit the pillow that night knowing that I stayed within my calorie budget. I remember the stress of that day, I remember my near meltdown in the drive-thru, but I can't recall if I exercised that day or not. It's not mentioned in the blog posting from Day Sixty, but my focus was clearly on just surviving at that point. If I made it to bed without having a complete meltdown gorge fest, I was satisfied.

The next morning, all was better. I dodged a bullet and learned a very valuable lesson. *I wasn't invincible.* Up to that point, having lost fifty-seven pounds in the first fifty-nine days, I was feeling pretty much unstoppable. I was seriously over-confident and really needed to face a day like sixty to really flex the muscle of this thing I called the Steel Curtain Zone. It was sheer determination to succeed, and I just couldn't fail this time. It just wasn't an option.

It's easy to stay on track when everything is seemingly perfect. The real test for me was surviving a serious storm of stress and emotions, without the comfort food provided. Instead, my comfort was found in victory over my natural tendencies to use and abuse food. The results were coming very quickly, and they were, because of my consistency and complete dedication to change. My comfort was no longer found in a binge. Now, my comfort was found in the thoughts and dreams of where I was headed along this road. All of which depended on my consistency and unwavering dedication to learning all about myself and what it really takes to lose weight successfully.

I was discovering truths that I had never given thought. I was discovering that I wasn't a victim, this morbid obesity wasn't a hopeless situation, and that I had a power that had been untapped my entire life. I had the power to throw away every excuse that ever held me back. I could completely let go and live happily, while I consumed less and exercised. Instead of greeting each day with dread, I was actually thrilled to be so wonderfully alive. It was quite possibly the most powerful thing I had ever experienced.

Section Six

Breaking Free

"The truth set me FREE!"

Chapter Thirty-One

Passion Turns the Key

O ne of the emotional problems I had experienced in the past revolved around a sense of loss over food. I was feeling like I was missing out on something, feeling lost, and longing for a reunion with my old consumption habits. Suddenly, I realized, that food was something I will always enjoy. I can and will, and do enjoy, in fact, I love food, and that's completely normal. It was an epiphany like no other, when I realized that food wasn't leaving me and I *wasn't* leaving food.

Food and I were simply redefining our relationship. I was no longer being an abuser of food. The thought that there is nothing I can't enjoy in a reasonable portion is comforting. I don't have to eat everything or all of it in one sitting; it will still be something I can enjoy, *reasonably,* tomorrow, or next week, or who knows when? But someday I just might enjoy a small piece of the most delicious cheesecake in the world, and that's all right and good.

Learning how to be an intuitive eater instead of an emotional eater, thus changing my relationship with food, was an amazing process. It really didn't take long, it just took a shift in my perspective. My life of obesity was like a math student who couldn't "get it," until one day they do, and then they "see it" differently the rest of their life. This passionate discovery was something that I just couldn't keep quiet about. I had to share what I was discovering. And yes, I know many before me had discovered it long before, but for me—all of a sudden, I could speak and understand their language. I could do their "math."

The passion for this change consumed me and oozed out of me whenever I would speak about it or write a blog post. I couldn't help it. As the weight loss started becoming more noticeable, the questions started coming every day. *How are you doing it?* And off I would go, speaking passionately about everything I believed, like a preacher in front of his congregation. It didn't matter where I was. In a convenience store, at Wal-Mart in the frozen foods section, or standing in a parking lot speaking to someone several cars away, I was always willing to share. It really made my day longer because suddenly a simple run to the store for a few items would turn into an hour-long weight loss discussion and seminar.

I didn't realize that speaking and writing about weight loss would become something I would do forever, until I was asked to speak at a kick-off event for a weight loss competition organized by Ponca City Medical Center. I had already shed the first hundred pounds when the hospital came calling on the radio station to help promote the entire "Lose to Win" program. It was perfect for me. I was asked to attend the marketing meeting and help organize the radio campaign. During the meeting, Bill revealed my weight loss success, and of course I started explaining, and after a few minutes worth of epiphany wielding passion, they overwhelmingly agreed that they wanted me to be the featured speaker at their kick-off event. I, of course, accepted the challenge, and proceeded to write and produce commercials that would help fill the room with people.

On February 19th, 2009, 417 people packed into a room with only 400 seats. The room was actually the cafeteria in the hospital basement, and it was a perfect setting and audience for my very first weight loss public speaking experience. Cathy Cole, the director of the program, had a few introductory words and then introduced me. Prior to the event, I was asked to speak for ten minutes, then, right before, I was asked to speak for twenty minutes. I agreed, but was really nervous about speaking for so long, *twenty minutes? That's a really long time! How would I ever fill so much time?* I ended up speaking for nearly forty minutes. How? *Pure passion, my friend.*

The energy in the room was electric and contagious. I approached the audience like I had done hundreds of times before as a stand-up comic, with a few laughs at the beginning, and then straight into my story, and what I was learning along the way. It was magical to me. A roller coaster of emotions swept across the room. Laughter, tears, serious looks from people listening intently, and the most amazing thing to me, was how naturally it all flowed. I didn't prepare a "set." This wasn't stand-up, this was the most "real" I had ever been in front of an audience. This was my first time to speak about weight loss, but I knew immediately, that speaking about weight loss was something I wanted to do for the rest of my life.

Something amazing happened that night. People became inspired, people talked about that night with their friends, co-workers, and who knows who else. All I know is, within three days, that standing room only crowd of 417 had swelled to over 800 participants in the program. Eight hundred people who really wanted to lose weight and choose change. In a town of only twenty-five thousand people, this was unheard of numbers. The program had more participants than other communities with upwards of one hundred thousand people. And the weight loss numbers were remarkable, with over seventy-five percent sticking with the program until the very end, compared to roughly twenty-five percent in other similar programs around the country.

I can't take a hundred percent credit for those numbers, but I do take pride in being on the team that had this much success, in such a dramatic fashion. It was an amazing effort by everyone involved, and life changing for some, no doubt.

It was certainly life changing to me. I was certain at that moment, that night, February 19th, 2009, that my future was pretty much decided. All of my experience in stand-up and broadcasting was just preparation for later. I was honing the skills that had most everything but a passionate message. Now, it had a passionate message. How could I experience the freedoms these weight loss truths were giving me, and not talk about it? I had to share, I had to try, I wanted to talk with every morbidly obese person in the world and personally tell them, *there is a way out!*

I spent years trying to figure out the seemingly "secret" message that Billy Gardell shared with me about my stand-up. I never forgot what he told me: *"If you ever figure out how much the audience really likes you, it will be like turning a key."* Billy was telling me to be myself, be real and passionate, and realize I already had the approval of the audience. Finding my passion and introducing the real me, a passionate me, was *like turning a key.*

I was filled with excitement about the future like never before. My blog continued stronger than ever, even though I really didn't have that many readers until sometime after Day Two Hundred. But it was never really about the number of readers. I was writing the blog for me. This was still my lifeline, my education about me, *from me.* I was still learning, and I still do today. As new readers would find me, I would suggest they read from Day One, and often times they did. What started happening next was something most unexpected and exciting.

I started getting emails from people who had read every single day and now they were managing their very own Calorie Bank and Trust! They were having success too and they were thanking me for writing the blog. Honestly, I was getting a little overwhelmed by it all. If the blog was important to me before, it just became important to me, times ten. When it started to really interfere with family activities or my sleep schedule, that's when I would say it became too much of a good thing for me. I was becoming addicted to the feedback from readers. And then I had to stop and ask myself a very important question.

Was I writing the blog for me? My daughters? Or was I writing it for people all over the world who would log in and read every day? Ultimately, it had to be for me and mine, and I tried very hard to make it that way. I was a long way from the goal and the daily writing continued like clock-work. Sharing my story in hopes of inspiring others would come naturally, it's who I was, it's what I do. *It's my passion.* But anything that threatened my success from developing in a pure and natural fashion couldn't be allowed. My obsession with sharing daily and getting that feedback instantly started shifting the important reasons for my blog in the first place.

Later, in August of 2010, I started missing regular daily post. It was one of the toughest things for me to do. For over twenty-two months, I had invested anywhere from one to three hours a night, seven days a week, writing the blog that was helping save my life. Backing off just a bit was probably a smart thing to do.

Chapter Thirty-Two

Another Stage

By the summer of 2009, I was feeling a confidence like I had never felt. I was looking in the mirror and for the first time in my life, and I was actually liking what I was seeing. My entire life I had felt like the most hideously obese and ugly person in every room I stood. But not anymore. I was transforming into the man I always wanted to be, the man I was supposed to be, the person I dreamed of becoming. And with that came pursuits that I felt were reserved for a fortunate few.

Just as I had discovered the power of being myself, I realized I felt enough like other people, maybe I could portray one. I had always dreamed of having a lead role in a stage play. Remember my role as a reporter in that school play years ago? Yeah, where my childhood obesity was the punch line, well—this time I was determined that it would be remarkably different. Auditions were coming up for the Regional Actors Community Theater's production "Call Me Henry." It wasn't a musical, which was a good thing. I wanted to act, not sing. So I marked it on the calendar and almost backed out at the last minute.

I was scared. *What if I failed? What if I couldn't act?* I had lost nearly 200 pounds at that point, but I was still kind of a big guy. Maybe I hadn't lost enough weight to pursue this type of thing. I realized at the last minute that I had to do it, I didn't have a choice. If I hadn't, I would have been seriously disappointed in myself. *Oh, my, I was so nervous.*

All of the actors auditioned in a big group, each taking turns front and center. The exercise I later learned was what convinced director Chris Williams to cast me. It was very interesting. We were each given a random newspaper article. Chris then asked each of us to read our stories and while we were reading he would direct our emotions. If Chris said sad, you had to reflect that in your reading. If he said excited or happy, then the reading needed to reflect the emotion. And when he shouted, "Anger!" I cut loose. I read that innocent little story about a fancy new softball complex being built near Tulsa, like they had stolen my momma's house, kicked her to the curb, tore it down, and built those ball diamonds. I was angry and Chris Williams knew it. My aggressive reading came from a place very deep within me.

All of those years of feeling the way I did about myself. All of the anger and resentment I once harbored for myself and others, all of it came out. I was passionately releasing this anger all over that little league softball complex story. And I left the director and producer slightly surprised. That was it. I had the part. Show me to my trailer, please. *What? You mean we don't get trailers in community theater productions?*

I was on top of the world. When Chris called me and asked if I would be the male lead, oh, my, *yes, yes, yes!* It was seriously a dream come true. And something I doubt would have ever happened at over 500 pounds. Let's face it, I would have never even auditioned back then. I was out and about, doing things that I felt I couldn't do before.

Talk about a crazy-busy time. Full-time job, plus rehearsal five times a week, plus writing the blog every night, plus working out, plus everything else. It was fast paced and hectic to say the least. I was so busy; I hardly noticed my family crumbling around me.

Chapter Thirty-Three

Letting Go Without Binging

I came home one afternoon, in a hurry, because I needed to drive to Blackwell and pay a bill before five o'clock, when Amber, home for the summer, asked if she could ride along. It wasn't necessarily unusual that she wanted to spend time with me, but something did seem different. Like there was another reason she wanted to ride along. And there was.

She told me that Mom was seeing someone else and that she and Courtney had discovered and confirmed what was happening. I was stunned, but not surprised. I looked at all we had been through and realized that despite my dramatic weight loss, it wasn't going to be enough to close the gap we each had inside ourselves. Holes in each other that refused to heal, issues that drove us each to do what we did, without concern for the consequences. Some might say we grew apart, others might interpret it very differently, but whatever the conclusion, it was a very sad moment. Irene certainly doesn't deserve all of the blame. We each played a role in our unfortunate demise.

We tried to work out our differences with counseling, but it just wasn't taking hold. In November 2009, right before Thanksgiving, we separated. On May 25th, 2010, we were officially divorced. It was a very sad ending to a twenty-one-year marriage. We left each other with mutual love and respect. We're still friends, and always will be. And most importantly, we'll always be the loving parents of Amber and Courtney.

We both needed forgiveness. I've forgiven Irene, but would she forgive me?

Irene is a woman who profoundly changed my life, saved my life figuratively and literally, in different ways. She was my caregiver, my love, one of the few people in my life that never, not even for a second, stopped believing in me. Her unyielding support of me often surpassed her best interest. *And how did I repay her?* By taking advantage and for granted her love and care. At my worst, when I was struggling with raging sleep apnea, urinating all over our bed in my disturbed sleep, and constantly depending on her to keep my swollen right leg manageable, she still loved me. Her actions displayed the most precious love one could ever hope to receive. To lift myself up, out of that horrible existence, was something that may not have ever happened without her incredible actions of love. For that I have an endless love and gratitude for her.

It doesn't seem fitting for such a monumental change to occupy such a relatively short section of this book. It wouldn't be fair to go through and try to explain every single thing that ultimately contributed to the end of our marriage. Irene and I have talked extensively about the deep issues that we both brought into our relationship. These issues were seeded long before we met in the halls of Stillwater High School. We've both forgiven one another for any negative effect we each had on our relationship, and we both recognize the amazing good we both contributed. Finally, we're both at peace with our lives before, during, and now after our twenty-two-year relationship. To attempt a deeper explanation wouldn't be correct in these pages.

I could have folded under the pressure of numerous circumstances throughout this transformation. The stress of a financial meltdown, marital issues, the extreme focus and attention I devoted to my writing, then the divorce, living single—dating, *oh, dear*. The Steel Curtain Zone was made for these events. Having a normal and healthy relationship with food couldn't be something that only happened when everything is perfect. Because life isn't perfect and *s*tress is a part of life. How we deal with stress is what separates. A wise person once said, life is twenty percent what happens to you and eighty percent how you respond. Attitude is everything. Emotional binging was a thing of the past, and the events along the way were proving this.

Through it all, I kept right on writing every single night, and working out almost every single day. My Steel Curtain Zone was in high gear, set to "extremely sensitive," as I navigated some of the hardest days of my life, with the calorie budget in great shape, and the scale continuing to drop the pounds. I wouldn't—I just couldn't— allow me or any person, place, thing, circumstance, or emotion change my behaviors with food. At the same time, I couldn't help noticing the tragic irony of the situation.

Going back to the night of September 13th, 2008, saving my family and keeping us together was the biggest motivator for me to begin along this road. Now, even though I was wildly successful at losing the weight, very different than any other attempt ever, we still crumbled. It was like we couldn't survive the changes on either side of the coin. If we could have just stayed the same as we had always been, then maybe we would still be together. But change was coming one way or another. I was either going to die young at over 500 pounds, or I was going to lose the weight and live like never before. Both ways provided enough turbulence in our lives, to shake us up permanently.

As a family, at one point, we had lost over 500 pounds collectively. Irene lost 140, Courtney lost 80, Amber 60, and over 200 pounds for me. It was an accomplishment that was far from complete for all of us individually, but still extremely impressive. The four of us, to this day, still feel an amazing family bond when we're all together. I imagine that will never change, regardless of who Irene or I call "honey." As long as we never call another person "buddy." That was ours. And we'll never have another buddy, like we had in each other.

Chapter Thirty-Four

Fitting In

In the middle of everything, my role in the play, and the beginning of the end for our family, as we knew it, I hit the two-hundred-pounds-lost milestone. I did it on Wednesday, August 5th, 2009. Two hundred one pounds lost in ten and a half months. It was a very amazing feeling. If I ever had any doubt before about reaching my goal, it was all gone now. I was headed straight to my goal weight of 230 pounds.

Some people criticized me for losing 200 pounds too fast, but really, if I'm eating well and I'm exercising, and most importantly, I'm doing it consistently every day, then *where's* the problem? Could I have lost it slower? Sure, probably, but how? By being inconsistent? By eating more than I needed? It's important to remember that the weight flies off in the very beginning, especially on someone as large as me. And as I got closer to that milestone, I started slowing down considerably. The lowest two week loss up until that point was five pounds. The very next weigh-in showed only a three pound loss. So, it is one and a half pounds a week. That doesn't sound unreasonable now, does it?

This entire transformation is like a bunch of dreams coming true all at once, with an occasional nightmare thrown in for balance, I guess. Before our separation and eventual divorce, we all did something I had looked forward to doing for years. On September 26th, 2009 it happened. And we were all together for the momentous occasion. You see . . .

We had taken the girls to Frontier City theme park several times over the years. Working in radio, I'd often have access to free or almost free tickets most every season. And it was always the same. I would walk around and watch everyone have fun. I was the official purse holder and ride watcher. I was too obese to ride most everything, except the log ride. The log ride didn't have a bar to hold you in place. Every trip to Frontier City was miserable for me. People would stare, they knew—I wasn't fitting on the rides, I was just along to watch and eat eight-dollar hamburgers. Actually, I'm pretty sure we always resisted the outrageously expensive theme park food, except for maybe some Dippin' Dots. Oh, man, I love me some Dippin' Dots.

I've never been a "ride person," and not just because I was morbidly obese. I was scared of most rides, all because of a horrible experience I had as a four-year-old at the carnival in downtown Stillwater, behind Katz Department Store. Mom took me to the carnival and we were having a grand old time, until we decided to ride the Tilt-A-Whirl. I was fine at first, but then the motion became too much, my mouth filled with what was once my lunch, and I held it in for as long as I could, and then, with a forceful expulsion . . . *splash!* everywhere. The ride continued on, slinging my sickness all over the place, people were screaming in horror, and the loudest was my mom. She was desperately trying to get the ride operator's attention, yelling, "Stop the ride, stop the ride!" She kept trying, but our movement was probably creating a Doppler effect, so all he was hearing was, "Stop, the . . ." It really didn't matter because he wasn't listening; he was enjoying the entire scene. I seriously remember him laughing as we whizzed by, being jerked around in different directions. The ride didn't stop until it was finished. And the ride man didn't even ask if I was alright. He just grabbed the hose and sprayed everything down. It must happen all the time because, seriously, they keep a hose ready. Who decided this was some kind of fun ride, anyway? I spent the next thirty-three years deathly afraid of any ride that might create the same situation as the Tilt-A-Whirl. But nothing, no fear, not a thing, was going to stop me from riding everything at Frontier City on that cool September Saturday.

After 213 pounds of weight loss, I had earned every ride. So on the way in, we all passed around the Dramamine tablets, reminiscent of the days when we would pass around the Zantac bottle after a heavy meal. This time, we were prepared to have a blast. I was still slightly scared, but I decided, sick or not, it didn't matter. I was joyously riding everything I could fit on and in. I was going to hear the easy "click" of every safety bar, *"Here—take it off, and do it again, I like that sound!"* Yes, it was an absolutely incredible experience. We took some awesome pictures that day, and I even recorded some video on my first roller coaster ride, as Irene and the girls told me to "put it away!"

"I made it! I did it and I didn't throw up! Let's do it again!" All of a sudden I was a kid again, but this time I wasn't afraid of anything. *I rode 'em all.* Even the coaster where your legs dangle in the breeze. That didn't scare me one bit. I was addicted to the "click" of that safety bar. Ride after ride, fitting perfectly and sharing this fun experience with my family, was one of the most memorable days of my life. I'll never forget the feeling I experienced that day. It was sweet freedom, made possible by my life-saving weight loss, or my, "dream come true making weight loss." I couldn't help but notice a couple of morbidly obese people at the amusement park that day, walking around, holding bags, and watching everyone have fun. I know exactly how they were feeling. I wondered if they ever dreamed of life being different. I wonder if they even thought it was possible. It was, and is, because I was living proof that day.

Chapter Thirty-Five

My Tools

My tools do not include pills, surgery, special meal plans, meal replacement products, weight loss center type plans, or special exercise equipment. My tools cannot be ordered from a late-night infomercial promising big results. You will not find them on any shelf in any store. This entire transformation never cost me a dime. In fact, I've actually saved money in several different ways.

The tools of my transformation are ones that I've had the entire time, I just never gave myself the power to tap their usefulness. I had to become the mechanic of my transformation, grabbing those tools and using them for the first time in my life. My instruction manual was self-honesty. When I fully embraced the truth about my abusive behaviors with food, regardless of how hard it was to accept and how horrible the truth hurt, it was like shining a bright light on every other weight loss attempt in my past. The shortcomings were obvious in the glaring light of truth. *The truth set me free.*

If you've skimmed over the story so far (I hope not), now isn't the time to skim. If the only thing you're interested in is the "how," I'm about to get to the mechanics of it all. If you haven't had your perspective shifted just yet, this chapter just might change the way you look at weight loss, forever. The "Emotion Ocean and Mix Tape of Our Mind," "The Long Answer to How?" and my favorite, "The Wrong Battle" just might give you some epiphanies that will leave you giddy for success and completely confident in your ability to succeed.

The mental dynamics really play the biggest role. On the three hundred twenty-seventh day, I sat down and wrote what I believe to be one of the most important pages in my entire blog archive.

I realize that talking about the mental changes being eighty percent of this battle, and talking about all of the little and big psychological gymnastics I've practiced to stay consistent, well, it just doesn't go deep enough. So take a big breath and let's go diving into the deep waters of our emotion ocean.

I've always had a fear of not living up to my potential. Never following through. Never becoming what my teachers, family, co-workers, coaches, and comedy colleagues just knew I could be. Potential. *Do I fear my potential?* Or do I fear *not living up to that potential* that everyone is so certain I hold within?

I've never had a problem convincing people to believe in me, but I've had a devil of a time convincing me to believe in myself. It's like I've had a mix tape playing over and over in my head for so many years. That mix tape would say horrible things to me, and it made me believe them.

You'll never live up to your potential. You'll always be fat and ugly. You'll never realize any professional success in broadcasting beyond a small market level. You'll pass your horrible behaviors with food onto your children. You're worthless and not worthy of success. Who do you really think you are? You're just a poor kid from the projects that will never amount to anything special. And you're stupid, an uneducated buffoon just faking his way through life, trying to convince everyone that you really have a clue.

What does the mix tape in your brain say every day to you?

I guess what I've done is this: I've hit the eject button on that old mix tape. Then, I destroyed it. It will never play in my mind again. Never. I've made a new mix tape. What I hear in my head every day now is this:

You will exceed your potential in ways you can't even fathom at this point. You will be healthy, thin, and handsome. Your success in broadcasting, motivational or inspirational speaking, and anything you decide you want to do is only limited by your imagination. Your example and guidance for your family is exemplary. Your worth is immeasurable and success is yours for the taking, go ahead, you deserve it. You are a man of integrity with amazing abilities of communication. You're a kid that was raised through humble beginnings completely surrounded by love and acceptance. You're a self-educated intelligent human being who doesn't have to convince anyone of anything.

Big difference, huh?

What we tell ourselves every day *is what we become.* It's true, my friend. *So why after a lifetime of fighting obesity am I breaking free so wonderfully now?* Because I destroyed that old tape and replaced it with something worthy of listening.

How do you make a new mix tape for your brain?

Write it out, memorize it, burn it into your brain, and most importantly . . . *believe* it.

Maybe it's too much to replace everything all at once. Replace one at a time, transform how you think about yourself at whatever pace you're comfortable.

Your old mix tape was made over time. It is the product of your past. And if you continue allowing the past to determine your future, then you'll always get the same result. Don't allow your past to own you—OWN IT. Put it in its place. Let the past know that its effects on your future are over right now. Don't try to completely forget about the past.

A good friend of mine told me that "you can't amputate your past and walk freely into the future." Your past is your story. It's made you who you are today, good or bad. But you can immediately decide that it will no longer control your future. And someday, that complete story that is you can and will shine as a light of hope to others. Letting them know that anything is possible, anything at all.

You'll be extracting lessons and epiphanies from your past experiences as you proceed down this road. These lessons and epiphanies couldn't be seen or realized before because you were too wrapped up in the life and times. This crystal clarity that's provided by time and experience becomes exceptionally clear when you start owning your choices with self-honesty that bares everything inside you.

I honestly didn't know what I was doing when I started. But I was doing these things, accidentally stumbling upon epiphanies that would prove to be life changing for me. I've been "acting as if . . ."

I've acted as if I was a normal responsible eating individual. I've acted as if I was someone who cared about exercising. I've acted as if I was someone that could share my story and help others along the way.

Three very powerful words: *Acting as if.* Why are they so powerful?

Because you become whatever you put into your brain. When you're "acting as if," you're training your brain to accept and transform to what you desire to become. *And you will.*

So now you know where my resolve comes from. Now you know why my consistency level is unwavering. Now you know why I'm so passionate about sharing my story, my triumphs, and my struggles.

Is it perfect? No. I've said that many times along this road. It doesn't have to be perfect, my friend. Striving for perfection is the quickest detour to disappointment. But if we continue with a positive consistent effort, and we change the way we think about ourselves, then our success is practically guaranteed. You will not be able to stop it from happening. And don't be afraid of success. Go ahead, *you deserve it.*

And the great thing about weight loss success? It happens slowly over time, allowing you to adjust and get used to the new you. You're going to absolutely love it.

If someone wants to know specifics about "how," I start explaining . . .

Because I've decided. I've written before about making that Iron-Clad Decision, and it's that decision to succeed, that rock-solid commitment to consistency that has given me these incredible results. I found out that you have to give this journey an amazingly high priority. You have to make it one of the most important things you do. You have to defend your journey from anything and everything that might try to derail it. You have to protect it from yourself. I was always my own worst enemy, I understand that.

When you make it this important, it really makes it hard to rationalize bad choices, *you know what I mean?* As dramatic as it might sound, this is life and death stuff, my friend. And no matter if you have thirty pounds or 300 to lose, if you give it that "do or die" level of importance in your life, you're less likely to fail. But is it that easy? Just decide? *Really?* Make it important? What? *No.*

Along with my iron-clad decision, I decided to throw away every single misconception I had about weight loss. I knew I wanted long-term results; I really wanted to change. So I eliminated any plan that wasn't completely natural. I needed something I could do that would keep me thin the rest of my life. I needed to learn what a normal portion looked like. I didn't want a "meal replacement" type plan, or a pre-packaged food "weight loss center" type of plan. I knew those type of plans were simply a means to lose weight temporarily. These plans might be perfect for someone who isn't a food addict or compulsive or emotional eater, but for someone like me, they're temporary at best. I needed to confront my behaviors with food in everyday situations, and it had to be head on with real food *like everybody else eats.*

I then determined that nothing was off limits. I could eat anything I wanted, and *I mean, anything!* That element of my journey has been one of the keys to success because, if nothing is off limits, then I'll never feel deprived . . . and I'll never feel defeated because I enjoyed something that conventional weight loss wisdom says you can't have if you want to lose weight.

It's not the food, it's the portions. Counting calories was a natural choice for me. It's taught me about proper portions and it's forced me to make better choices along the way. I opened the Calorie Bank and Trust in my mind, treating my calories like cash. I quickly learned that good choices meant making wise calorie "investment" decisions. I had to spread those calories out all day long, or run short as a consequence. Remember what I said earlier, the Calorie Bank and Trust doesn't have an ATM. When the calories are gone, they're gone until the bank opens the next morning. It might sound silly, but it's not—look what it's done for me.

But those urges to binge, how do I control those nasty things? Those crazy thoughts that sometimes come from out of nowhere, stealing away my resolve, making me fantasize about eating large quantities of anything that I love, how have I handled them?

Motivating thoughts plus accountability plus writing out my thoughts every night. That's how I've handled those journey-breaking meltdowns. I tell anyone who cares to listen: *"Cling tight to those motivating thoughts, defend your journey like your life depends on it, in most cases it does. Decide that nothing . . . no emotion, no circumstance, no person, place or thing is allowed to steal this away from you. I deserve this success. You deserve this success. It's too important, my friend."*

One of the biggest elements is self-honesty. This means calling yourself on all those excuses and rationalizations that we tell ourselves in order to feel better about bad choices. Honesty, one hundred percent, *at all times.* And exercise? *Anything* . . . just move. All I could do in the beginning was walk and I could barely do that for very long. But I was moving. And the more you move, the easier it gets.

223

All of a sudden my 505-pound, near-deadly quarter-mile walks became a mile . . . then two, then three, and so on. In the beginning it doesn't have to be anything special. Just movement. After a while you can get fancy. But set a solid foundation for success first by mastering the basics.

I was having breakfast with Mom one morning at one of our favorite little diners, Shortcakes in Stillwater, when she expressed frustration and confusion over what to eat on any particular day. She was obviously struggling and completely stressed over her many food options. *"I just can't seem to make the right choices with the food, it's so hard sometimes."*

I knew that Mom's struggles really were not centered around her food choices, like she was convinced. Her struggle was with her tendency to be her own worst enemy. Her resolve to stay consistent, her iron-clad decision and the actions, and self-honesty required, were nearly non-existent. But it wasn't those things that she credited, or blamed, for her failure to stay on track and really lose weight. It was the food. Her battle was always focused on fighting food. Food was her enemy, food was evil, food, food, food! Why do we love it so much?

Because food is good. And food doesn't want to fight us. It never wanted to fight us. Food *is* simply wanting to nourish our bodies, giving us just what we need to be healthy. Food didn't ask to be abused by us. It's not food's fault that we abuse it, and as a result, abuse ourselves. Food *is* an ally. Food can be a wonderful friend. We just have to learn to be a better friend to ourselves and to food.

I kept talking to Mom that morning, over an egg white veggie omelet with hash brown potatoes, and the more I talked, the clearer my thought process became. Mom inspired me in that moment. I had to find a way to communicate this message in a way that couldn't be argued by any reasonable human. If you understand, then you too just might realize, that the following analogy is critical to process and understand. And once you do, you will never look at weight loss the same, and you will be armed with a new perspective that has the power to propel you to goals you thought were nearly impossible.

When I look back at my many failed weight loss attempts, I can clearly see a crucial error in my battle plan. This mistake was the reason for my yo-yo dieting. This mistake was why it was always a struggle every single day as I lost weight in the past. This flaw is one that is made by millions of others everyday along this road . . . it's the reason for the madness, it's the reason why we're conditioned to believe that weight loss is hard. *What is it?* Please read . . .

I was always fighting the *wrong* battle. I didn't know who or what was the real enemy. How can you effectively battle if you haven't identified the real enemy? I made food my enemy, that was the battle. I was always determined to put the food in its place. I would try to defeat food at every turn. Food wasn't going to win. That was my battle. The perceived enemy: *food.* But while I was busy battling food, the real enemy would sneak in from the side and defeat me every time in a battle that I didn't even realize I should be fighting. The real enemy? *Me.*

Food never wanted to fight me, food was my friend, my all, but I was convinced otherwise. It was food that made me fat, right? NO. I made me fat by using and abusing my friend in food. But I could never admit that before. So the battle with my perceived enemy of food would continue. I'd make special lists, set portion sizes, count those calories, resist temptation at every turn, battle it, fight with everything I had, but in the end I would always lose the fight. Why? How?

Wait just a second. Once again, this sounds like what I've done, but wait . . . it wasn't and isn't the same.

What ended my past weight loss battles? It wasn't food. It was the real enemy: *Me.* Armed with excuses, rationalizations, and slinging blame wherever I could, the real enemy would show up on the scene and completely stop me in my tracks. Even if I had lost 115 pounds like I did in 2004, the real enemy would step in and take it all back, plus some, and it happened time and time again.

And it happened because I was fighting the wrong enemy. I was waging war on an ally, whose only desire was to be my friend. No wonder I failed so many times at losing weight! It wasn't until this time, when I discovered the power of self-honesty and hundred-percent self-responsibility in my behaviors with food, that the real battle became clear.

And now I know the real enemy. But the goal isn't and never has been to pummel this enemy. The goal has always been to turn this enemy into an ally. It's about becoming friends with *yourself*.

And that's what's happened over the course of this transformation road. I realized the enemy wasn't really food and that food was always my friend, and I realized, although I had always been my own worst enemy, I had the power to call a truce, with a self-honesty and responsibility pact that would leave me good friends with this former enemy . . . friends with food and friends with myself.

The needless battles are over. There's no peace in those battles. But here, oh, my, there's all kinds of wonderful peace and freedom. Freedom to live, breathe, eat, and continue down this road without the frustrations that always plagued my past weight loss attempts. When someone asks, *"So, you worried about gaining all that weight back?"* I smile and say, *"No, not at all."* It might sound over-confident to them, but when you haven't an enemy to battle, the fight is over and all that's left is gentle understanding and peace.

Chapter Thirty-Six

Facing My Biggest Bully

Two years, two months, and a day. That's how long it took. On November 16th, 2010, I hit the number I had my sites on from the very beginning—230 pounds.

I hit goal. *I hit GOAL!* I stepped onto the same scale where more than a dozen of my past attempts started, the same scale that weighed me 505 on Day Two now showed me 230.4 on seven hundred eight-ninth day. I've *always* rounded up or down. Had it been point five, I would've been two hundred thirty one. The bottom line: I was two hundred thirty pounds. *I did it.*

It was never just about the physical transformation. It was about a complete transformation of mind, body, and soul. If I truly wanted this time to be unlike any other previous attempt, I had to explore every molecule of who I was and who I am and what I will always be.

Along the way, I realized that certain non-food related issues needed to be resolved. I was experiencing a transformation of my mind, body, and soul, but still, I harbored negatives that had to be addressed before I could truly experience the kind of clarity I desired.

Inside my heart was anger and resentment for my father, whom I had met years earlier, but had remained estranged from for more than seventeen years. Now that things were changing in a positive direction, I needed to discover the true meaning of forgiveness. I needed to make my heart beat normally again.

I had never met my two half brothers, and that's something that I really wanted and needed to do. As for a relationship with my father? A positive relationship was critical for me, and him, too, I believe. I didn't want to someday find his obituary on the Internet, and then realize I didn't have another chance to know him in some way.

So, not too far down this road, I once again contacted my father. Since December of 2009, we've exchanged emails, phone calls, and he even occasionally reads my blog. He even spent the better part of a week with me at my home in June of 2010. After several wonderful conversations, his message to me was simple. He doesn't want me to live a life of regrets, but he wants me to excel, and leave no stone unturned on my journey to a wonderful life.

I made a trip to Alabama in November 2010 and stayed with my dad's sister, Aunt Beverly. I also had a chance to attend my grandfather's 88th birthday celebration, where I not only took a wonderful picture with him, but I had a chance to meet so many other family members I never knew. I was made to feel so welcomed. And Dad and I had a good visit, too.

It's amazing how wonderful our very simple relationship is now, after letting go of the past. I'm learning that my dad is a very real, very good person, and like all of us, he's struggled with good and bad choices. He understands that choosing to not be a part of my life was a mistake (or it might have been the best thing for both of us). Regardless of good or bad, it's one choice that he regrets deeply.

We're past all that now, and with the slate wiped clean with complete and total forgiveness, we can move forward to a mutually wonderful relationship. Experiencing real forgiveness was like an actual weight lifted from my heart. I was free to let it all go and simply live and love, *forever.*

I never got a chance to meet Danny, my older half brother. Before we could reconnect, he died from aortic dissection, the same condition that killed John Ritter, a condition caused by years of uncontrolled high blood pressure. He was forty-two. I still haven't met, but I've connected via telephone with my younger half brother, Silas. Perhaps someday we'll have a chance to meet face to face.

I may not have had the chance to meet Danny, but I met his beautiful, smart, wickedly funny and talented daughter, Kayla. Kayla and I hit it off immediately. We're two of a kind in so many ways. As a proud father of two daughters, I found myself naturally gravitating toward her, wanting to give her encouragement. I wanted her to know that she also has the power to rise up above everything and succeed beyond her wildest dreams.

These renewed and some brand new relationships were absolutely imperative to my development along this road. They are a vital part of my transformation on the inside.

When the thought processes that helped keep me safely over 500 pounds started to change, I started changing my habits without even trying. I was once addicted to internet poker sites. I would spend hours and hours playing in online tournaments, sometimes all night long on the weekends. I never played for big money; in fact, I once spent over six hours in front of the computer, doing really well in a tournament that cost me ten cents to enter, only to win a little over a dollar. When I started focusing on losing weight and writing my blog, I immediately stopped playing online poker. I didn't even miss it. I simply didn't have the time or energy for online poker.

There was a time when we were addicted to television. Mostly every night, we had our shows. American Idol, Deal or No Deal, Extreme Makeover, and several others I can't remember. We were dedicating hours upon hours every week to sitting and watching. Most of my habits included sitting and not moving much at all. As soon as the weight started dropping, the blog started, and all of a sudden I would go days, even weeks at a time without watching any television. None! I was way too busy! I didn't miss it either. It was months into my journey when I looked back and realized, hey, I hardly ever do that anymore. Just as my choices with food slowly evolved into better choices, my choices in almost every other part of my life improved as well, and in a very natural fashion.

I've talked extensively about overcoming emotional and compulsive eating, and finding control and balance as a food addict. Another of the critical elements of my success has been exercise. My exercise evolved fairly quick. On that first night, it was walking less than a quarter mile. Within a week, I was up to what I thought was a mile, but later found out was actually point eighty-six of a mile. And it wasn't long after that, I found myself inside the YMCA, using a membership that I had for so long (a wonderful benefit of working at Team Radio!) but I rarely used.

The YMCA was something special to me. It was a place full of positive energy. One of my favorite activities in the early days of my weight loss was to play racquetball against the wall. Trying to keep up with the ball was the challenge that was wearing me out every time. It was an amazing workout. And like everything else, as I progressed, it became easier and easier.

Going back into the YMCA was kind of tough at first. Not the workout, but facing the director, Shane Harland. Shane was one that cheered me on back in 2004 as I lost 115 pounds, so coming back with all of that weight back on, was especially tough. I hated feeling like I disappointed him. He, along with Stephanie Williams and everyone else at the YMCA, has always been so incredible to me. The one thing that hasn't changed is my profile picture on the YMCA computer system. It's still the 500-pound Sean. I love it when I check in and my picture comes up, especially if it's someone brand new because they always do a double take. Sometimes they even ask me about the weight loss, or I hear them asking someone else about the picture.

It took me a little while to get over being self-conscious at the YMCA. I'm still a little self-conscious, but in the beginning, I was, *extremely* self-conscious. Inside that racquetball court, I felt like a zoo animal on display. I realize now that these stories I created in my head were completely opposite to what most everyone was thinking. Instead of *"Oh, my, look at that guy"* it was, *"Wow, look at him go, very nice. Glad he's here and working out, that's awesome."* It wasn't easy convincing myself of that truth, but after awhile, I just didn't allow the negative thoughts to enter. I was there and I was doing positive things for myself with every visit. The coolest thing was how people would notice and comment on my progress. Talk about motivating, supportive, and inspiring, that place, wow. They're just incredible and an amazing benefit to me.

One of the things I often hear from people is, *"I just can't exercise."* Physically, they have convinced themselves it's impossible. If that's you, prove yourself wrong. And this is how: Start very small. Just walk fifty feet or so. Do it again the next day. Every day, try to go just a little further. This is exactly the approach I had to take. I was scared that if I tried anything too tough, I would drop dead! Keep it simple and keep moving, every day. You'll amaze yourself by how quickly you'll develop. You might be a marathon runner someday, seriously. I know you might not be able to imagine that now, but you'll see, you'll absolutely see.

One of the most memorable nights along this entire road was the night Courtney was standing in the hall of our home and ripping to shreds a girdle that held her captive for years. I was so moved by her emotional and physical freedom that I asked for her permission to write about her experience. She agreed and I immediately erased whatever it was I was starting to write that night. There wasn't anything more important than this, there still isn't:

Once there was a little girl of eleven years old who was searching for something to make her feel better about her appearance. Her extra weight was wreaking havoc on her self-image and her confidence was at horribly low levels. She started looking for outfits that would "slim," and became very particular about what she would and wouldn't wear.

Then one day she discovered something that promised to tighten, slenderize, and magically improve her appearance. All she had to do was wear it every day underneath her clothes. She started wearing this magical garment without telling her parents. In her mind it made all the difference in the world. It wasn't long before she became addicted.

It was her secret garment. Not even her friends knew what she was wearing underneath. Wearing this undergarment required some extreme discipline and abuse to her body, for when she had it on, she couldn't easily go to the bathroom. So all through the sixth grade she held in any urge she had to use the restroom. Not once did she ever go to the bathroom, unless it was to check her appearance in the mirror.

When her parents finally discovered this undergarment and realized how restrictive and possibly damaging it could be, they ordered it off and discarded. This did not go over well with this beautiful little girl. Her reaction was one of tears and screams, like they had just ripped her whole world out from under her.

She convinced her parents that if she really had to use the restroom, she wouldn't let this undergarment get in the way, and they allowed the undergarment to stay in her possession, protecting her self-image like a bullet-proof vest.

Her obsession continued through the sixth, seventh, eighth, ninth, and even tenth grade. Not one bathroom break in over four and a half years of school days. That is until a month ago.

That's when this beautiful little girl, now fifteen years old, took it off for good. Her weight loss success has made the undergarment completely useless. Her smaller size has rendered that "magical" garment powerless. She no longer needs that girdle to give her a boost of confidence about her appearance. Exercise and good calorie management has swooped in and really made some serious changes in her body and most importantly, in her mind.

But she couldn't throw it away, what if she needed it again? So she hid it away. That little girl is my youngest daughter, Courtney.

Tonight Courtney finally convinced herself she would never need it again, so she pulled out that old girdle and started ripping it apart. We then took it one step further, walked out on our patio and lit it on fire. Tonight that girdle burned.

It burned almost as bright as Courtney's new-found confidence and self-image.

Amber left for college in the fall of 2008, shortly before I started losing weight. My blog was a way for me to connect with her on a very deep level. I believe we have that connection now more than ever. Her love and compassion for helping children with developmental disabilities is making her an absolute superstar in my eyes. She has an amazing gift inside her. And I feel confident that she knows, the sky is the limit. Her bounds are dictated only by her imagination and dreams. Both of my daughters realize that they can do anything they set their minds to.

I'll always be there for Amber and Courtney, and so many others that I love.

Irene will always have a special place in my heart. Despite anything and everything that we put ourselves and each other through, we still have love, understanding, and forgiveness for each other. We lived an absolutely amazing life together. Not easy, but unbelievably amazing on many different levels. And we'll always be the two best parents we can be to Amber and Courtney.

I spent the first thirty-six years of my life believing, if I'd never been overweight, I would have sailed through life without a single problem. I don't believe that anymore.

Every now and again, something triggers certain emotions. It's like the world is doing its best impression of Clint Eastwood, not a word, just a look, as it sizes me up before unleashing a powerful kick to my shin. I might still flinch or even fall to the ground occasionally, but now I know how to get back up, dust myself off, and hold my head high. What I will not do is join in and continue to kick myself over and over. I will fight back when necessary. I will stand up for myself, even if it's against my toughest bully . . . *Me.*

If you want to change, approach your desire with complete self-honesty and integrity. Facing the truth, *the real truth,* is a component that cannot be overlooked. Don't over-complicate the process. If you're complicating the process, you're making it hard. Get extremely real with yourself and realize that you have the power to choose change before change chooses you. Because change is coming, one way or another, and God willing, it might as well be on your terms. Nothing ever stays the same. Good or bad, we're always transforming. We have the power to make it a most wonderful transformation.

Good Choices,
Sean A. Anderson

Resources

www.calorieking.com
Calorie King also publishes a book. This website was a wonderful tool for me along the way.

Www.myfitnesspal.com
I haven't used this service personally—but I know many people who have and love it!

Www.milestonesprogram.org
Dr. Marty Lerner Ph.D heads one of the most highly regarded eating disorder programs in the World in South Florida

Www.oa.org
Overeaters Anonymous is an amazing program that's helped millions around the globe.

Www.tops.org
TOPS stands for Taking Off Pounds Sensibly and I'm all about that! I actually attended a few meetings as a pre-teen and although I'm not a member today, TOPS is one of the few organizations I fully recommend for wonderful support along this road.

Www.weightwatchers.com
I've never been a member of Weight Watchers, but I'm friends with many successful WW members. Weight Watchers is one of the few heavyweights in the weight loss industry I actually respect and admire. Great program!

Www.lifecoachgerri.com
Gerri Helms is more than a friend, she's my life coach!

Www.jackfit.blogspot.com
A self-descibed "healthy living blogger," but most of us know Jack as the World's premier weight loss comedy blogger. Get ready to laugh out loud, every time you stop by his site.

Www.theantijared.com
Tony Posnanski –221 Pound loser and a no-nonsense weight loss blogger with a heart of gold and a fabulous story.

Www.mizfitonline.com
Carla Birnburg is an award winning writer, personal trainer, bodybuilder, and someone who started blogging before anyone even knew the word "blog."

www.keepingthepoundsoff.com
Jane Cartelli has lost over 200 pounds—on her impressive blog, she relates how she has and continues to do something that once seemed impossible, she's keeping the pounds off! A great blog for those recovering from food addiction, like me!

Www.hungrygirl.com
Lisa Lillien has made a successful career out of getting the best value out of every calorie—writing and sharing it all along the way! She has some amazing books too!

Www.greatday.com
Ralph Marston is one of my favorite modern day philosophers. His writings often have a timeless and universal truth that can't be denied or ignored, for too long.

Www.whoatemyblog.com
After starting his weight loss journey at 632 pounds, Stephen Vinson is on target to lose over 400 and he's blogging all the way there and beyond!
Www.transformationroad.com
My home on the internet with a link to my blog, facebook, and twitter! And of course, you can always contact me here: sean@transformationroad.com

www.losingweighteveryday.blogspot.com
The Daily Diary of a Winning Loser –This is the blog that started it all for me. I encourage you to go into the archives and read from Day 1 for a complete perspective of my entire weight loss journey.

www.facebook.com/transformationroad
Now that you've read the book, please share your reviews, thoughts, and comments on the official "Transformation Road" Facebook page

CPSIA information can be obtained at www.ICGtesting.com
Printed in the USA
LVOW102218020112

262083LV00008BA/195/P